AYURVEDA COOKBOOK

A STARTING PATH TOWARDS AYURVEDIC LIFESTYLE BY FEEDING YOUR BODY AND NOURISHING YOUR SOUL

ALISSON POT

© COPYRIGHT 2019 BY ALISSON POT ALL RIGHTS RESERVED

This document is geared towards providing exact and reliable information in regards to the topic and issue covered. The publication is sold with the idea that the publisher is not required to render accounting, officially permitted, or otherwise, qualified services. If advice is necessary, legal or professional, a practiced individual in the profession should be ordered.

- From a Declaration of Principles which was accepted and approved equally by a Committee of the American Bar Association and a Committee of Publishers and Associations.

In no way is, it legal to reproduce, duplicate, or transmit any part of this document in either electronic means or printed format. Recording of this publication is strictly prohibited and any storage of this document is not allowed unless with written permission from the publisher. All rights reserved.

The information provided herein is stated to be truthful and consistent, in that any liability, in terms of inattention or otherwise, by any usage or abuse of any policies, processes, or directions contained within is the solitary and utter responsibility of the recipient reader. Under no circumstances will any legal responsibility or blame be held against the publisher for any reparation, damages, or monetary loss due to the information herein, either directly or indirectly.

Respective authors own all copyrights not held by the publisher.

The information herein is offered for informational purposes solely and is universal as so. The presentation of the information is without contract or any type of guarantee assurance.

The trademarks that are used are without any consent and the publication of the trademark is without permission or backing by the trademark owner. All trademarks and brands within this book are for clarifying purposes only and are owned by the owners themselves, not affiliated with this document.

DISCLAIMER

The information contained within this eBook is strictly for educational purposes. If you wish to apply ideas contained in this eBook, you are taking full responsibility for your actions.

The author has made every effort to ensure the accuracy of the information within this book was correct at time of publication. The author does not assume and hereby disclaims any liability to any party for any loss, damage, or disruption caused by errors or omissions, whether such errors or omissions result from accident, negligence, or any other cause.

Table of Contents

Introduction 1

Chapter 1: Ayurveda: Body, Mind, And Soul 17

    The Universe And How We Are Connected 18

    The Five Elements: Building Blocks Of Nature 21

    The Three Doshas: Vata, Pitta, And Kapha 28

    The Twenty Qualities: An Important Key To Healing 36

Chapter 2: How We Can Stay Health y 42

    A Simple Home Purification 55

    Rejuvenation And Rebuilding 60

    Three Cautions About Home Panchakarma 62

    Ayurvedic Lifestyle: The Ultimate Preventive Medicine 66

    Ayurvedic Daily Routine 69

    Best Oils By Body Type 79

    Seasonal Routines 91

    Guidelines For Summer 92

Guidelines For Fall 99

Guidelines For Winter... 104

Guidelines For Spring.. 110

Ayurvedic Dietary Guidelines.. 114

Food Guidelines For The Constitutional Types.......... 115

Food Guidelines For The Basic Constitutional Types... 121

The Six Tastes.. 121

Effects Of Tastes On The Doshas.................................. 129

Eating Habits To Cultivate... 133

Unhealthy Eating Habits 135

Incompatible Food Combinations................................ 136

Recommendations Regarding Milk And Milk Products 139

Food And The Three Gunas.. 141

Psychological Constitutions.. 142

Relationship Of The Gunas And The Doshas............... 148

Chapter 3: Ayurveda's Staple Food....................... 150

Simple Ayurvedic Recipe: A Recipe For Flexible Cooking 151

How To Cook For The Doshas (And Agni) 152

How To Modify Your Cooking For Doshas And Agni 154

Chapter 4: Ayurveda Recipes 163

1. Ayurvedic Falafel 165

2. Ayurvedic Sauerkraut (Homemade Pickled Cucumber) 169

3. Healing Turmeric Smoothie 172

4. Ayurvedic Oatmeal 173

5. Ayurvedic Rose Smoothie 175

6. Chile-Garlic Potatoes And Cauliflower With Turmeric 178

7. Ayurvedic Garam Masala 181

8. Ginger Elixir (An Ayurvedic Digestive Drink) 184

9. Ayurvedic Spinach-Mung Detox Soup 186

10. Kitchari – The Nutritious Ayurvedic Detox Dish .. 189

Chapter 5: Ayurvedic Food Combining 196

A Balanced Approach To Food Combining 198

Combinations To Reduce Or Avoid 200

Introduction

While ayurveda, India's indigenous health system, is a vast and ancient subject, much of its common-sense wisdom is applicable today. My favorite thing about Ayurveda is the central role that food plays in well-being. Whether you like to cook or not, food medicine for the mind, and a little intention in your diet can truly change your perspective on life. Harmonizing the energies of the mind can relieve stress, increase joy, and foster spiritual connection. What's not to love?

To ensure success, be keeping our discussion simple in both theory and practice. You don't have to read this book cover to cover to benefit from the recipes, but it never hurts to have a clear road map for the journey. This brief introduction will set the stage for our exploration of the mind, how food affects the mind, and how you can apply Ayurveda in your own life to create mental balance.

the origins of ayurveda

Ayurveda (pronounced "EYE-yer-VAY-da") may be the oldest continually practiced health system in the world, dating from two thousand to five thousand years ago. The earliest information on Ayurveda is contained in the Rig Veda, one of four bodies of ancient scripture that were orally transmitted in lyrical phrases called sutras (threads). The Vedas are believed to originate from the rishis, sages in deep states of meditation.

Ayurveda can be loosely translated as the "science of life." The classical text the Charaka Samhita describes Ayur, or "life," as being made up of four parts: the physical body, the mind, the soul, and the senses (sight, hearing, touch, smell, and taste). Contrary to Western models, which have traditionally focused mostly on the physical body, Ayurveda has always given attention to the health of all four of the fundamental aspects of life. The system looks at the whole person—using diet, biorhythms, herbal medicine, psychology, wholesome lifestyle, surgery, and therapeutic bodywork to address the root cause of disease. Ayurvedic hospitals and clinics abound in India, where Western medicine is often used in conjunction with the traditional methods. Whereas Western medicine excels at resolving acute situations, Ayurveda stands out as a preventive medicine—seeking to halt the progression from imbalance to disease by addressing the underlying causes on.

THE BIG PICTURE

Ayurveda recognizes that every human being is a microcosm (a small part or reflection) of the macrocosm (the big picture or universe). Our minds and bodies are made up of the same elements that make up everything around us, and we are moved by the same energies or forces that move the oceans, the winds, the stars, and the planets.

The philosophy behind Ayurveda is simple: just as the cycles of the sun, moon, tides, and seasons ebb and flow, so do we. The introduction of artificial light, global food transportation, and a busy schedule make it easy to get out of sync with nature's rhythms.

Ayurveda and Yoga actually stem from the same philosophical roots and have a shared goal of creating a union between microcosm and macrocosm. Yoga is a pathway for navigating the connection of the mind and body with the larger world around us. The sattvic diet, sometimes called the yogic diet, is a part of this path. In these modern times, when many suffer in body and mind due to a lack of connection, the shared goal of Yoga and Ayurveda to unite mind, body, and spirit couldn't come at a better time. Ayurveda often uses the movements and breathing techniques from yoga to access the energy body, promoting the smooth circulation of energy throughout the body and mind, which is especially helpful for managing stress and restoring the body's natural rhythms.

If you get out of sync with natural rhythms—for example, by eating tropical fruits in winter or processed foods, staying up all night, or working all day without a break—your body and mind will become out of whack. The link between the mind and overall health is clear—imbalance in one will lead to imbalance in the other. Like a fish swimming upstream, going against natural currents will slow you down. Inevitably, you will start to feel tired, anxious, or depressed, and over time, you will end up "out of order."

THE POWER OF DIGESTION

Healthy digestion is the most fundamental aspect of overall wellness in Ayurveda. The complete digestion, absorption, and assimilation of food nutrients create the building blocks of the body, called ahara rasa, or "the essence of food." When you chew and swallow your food, it mixes with water, enzymes, and acids, and the end product is the essence or juice, which is used to make tissues. In this way, healthy digestion makes a healthy body. Digesting food properly connects us to the essence of the food we eat every day and to our planet that provides this food. This explains why diet is a profound aspect of Ayurvedic healing.

Complete wellness, however, takes into account not only physical digestion in the stomach, but mental digestion as well. The digestion of ideas, experiences, and emotions is a key function required for our overall well-being. The right amount of input and enough space to process it result in a calm, steady mind and nervous system.

This sustainable, low-stress reality underlies the health of the physical body as well. The body and mind are interdependent systems affected by parallel influences: the physical world of the five elements, and the energetic world of stillness, movement, and change. It can be easier to recognize tangible elements in the body first, so let's look at body basics before we dive into the topic of mind.

THE FIVE ELEMENTS

In Ayurveda, human anatomy starts with the five elements—ether (space), air, fire, water, and earth.

The elements create three compounds that govern specific functions and energies in the body, namely, movement, transformation, and cohesion (holding things together). According to Charaka, when these compounds, known as doshas, are in balance and working harmoniously, you will enjoy smooth-moving processes (digestion, circulation, and so on), clear senses, the proper elimination of wastes, and happiness.

Each of these five elements manifests as qualities in the body that can be recognized simply by paying close attention to physical sensations. For example, air and space are cold and light, fire is hot and sharp, and earth and water are heavy and moist. Imbalance is brought on by too much or too little of any of these qualities.

Too much dryness, say from living in the desert and eating dry crackers, will result in a symptom like dry skin. These elements can have corresponding effects on the mind, such as the heavy, moist qualities of earth and water resulting in brain fog, or the light, mobile qualities of air and space inhibiting focus. Ayurveda manages these imbalances by introducing opposite qualities and reducing similar qualities.

For example, in the case of brain fog, introducing light, dry foods like barley and reducing heavy, moist foods like wheat will begin to alleviate the symptom. Everyone requires all five elements, but they occur in different amounts in different bodies. Understanding your individual elemental makeup can take some time. By paying attention to your body over the course of changing seasons, you'll begin to recognize the major players. If dry skin, scalp, stool, and so on are a part of your world, it's likely there's a good deal of space and air elements in your body. Once this becomes clear, start feeling for the subtle qualities of these elements in your mind and moods. Space and air, for example, can manifest as an anxious, sometimes spacey, ungrounded, or sensitive mind or mood due to the porous nature of these elements.

While it is important to understand how Ayurveda views the physical body, in this book we will be looking mostly at the mind. Ayurveda considers the functions of body and mind to be so interconnected that balance and imbalance are rooted in both physical and mental spheres. It is important to our overall well-being to understand both.

What is a dosha?

You have probably heard of the doshas. According to the Ashtanga Hrdayam, dosha literally means "that which is faulty." But doshas aren't a problem until imbalance has been hanging around awhile. These energies, each a synergy of two elements, can hurt or help you, depending on whether or not they are in a relative state of balance.

That's why it is more important to understand how to maintain balance than it is to dwell on doshas as the "bad guys." There are three doshas, known as vata, pitta, and kapha. These are the compounds that arise naturally when the five elements come together in the human body. Each performs a specific function in the body and manifests as a recognizable group of qualities. While the primary energies that affect the mind are different from the three doshas, when one or more of the doshas accumulate in your body, you are likely to notice the same qualities in your mind.

Vata ("VA-tah") is the energy of movement.

Pitta ("PITT-ah") is the energy of transformation.

Kapha ("CUP-hah") is the energy of structure and lubrication together; cohesion (think glue).

VATA

Where there is space, air begins to move, and together these elements manifest as cold, light, dry, rough, mobile, erratic, and clear qualities. Think of vata as the currents of the body. The body knows the food goes in the mouth, then down and out; vata ushers it along. Vata also moves the attention and is responsible for the movements of the five senses and the activity of the brain and nervous system. The expansive nature of its qualities makes for a creative, mobile energy. There is nothing problematic about the qualities of space and air, or their function, unless your body has accumulated too much. Too many vata qualities can result in signs of imbalance such as gas and constipation, increasingly dry skin, and racing thoughts and anxiety.

PIT TA

Where there is fire, there has to be water to keep it from burning everything up. The resulting compound is firewater, a liquid, hot, sharp, penetrating, light, mobile, oily, smelly grouping of qualities. (Think acid or bile.) When food gets chewed, pitta moves in to break it down, liquidize it, metabolize it, and transform it into tissues.

It does the same with raw information, breaking it down, understanding it, and organizing it. The sharp, motivated nature of pitta makes for quick, focused energy. This is great, unless things get too hot or too sharp, resulting in signs of imbalance such as acidy burps or reflux; diarrhea; skin rashes; inflammation; or mental states that include irritability, obsession, and jealousy.

KAPHA

Without water, you wouldn't be able to get sand to stick together to build a sandcastle. The earth element requires water in this same way to get things to stick together. Kapha is like glue: cool, liquid, slimy, heavy, slow, dull, dense, and stable. This group of qualities provides density in the bones and fat, cohesion in the tissues and joints, and plenty of mucus so we don't dry out. Its gentle, soft, sticky nature makes for a mellow, sweet energy and a strong memory. Great! Unless things get too heavy and too sticky, which can result in signs of imbalance such as loss of appetite; slow digestion; sinus troubles and allergies; weight gain; or mental states

like heaviness, brain fog, and sadness.

In an ideal world, we would all have a decent dose of all of these qualities and a balanced, well-functioning system. One person may be more fiery and prone to arguments, another may be more spacey and prone to forget things—that's the fun of variation in nature. The body's constitution, or makeup of the elements, is genetic. Understanding your constitution can help you understand which of these compounds is likely to get out of balance so you can make choices in your diet and lifestyle to keep potential doshas in check.

It's easy to focus on dosha, that which gets out of balance. But categorizing yourself as a dosha ("I'm so vata") or identifying yourself with states of imbalance is not the aim of Ayurvedic wisdom. It may be more helpful to understand and manage the general causes of imbalance first. For instance, if you notice you often feel overheated and irritable, and your imbalances tend toward characteristics on the pitta list, practice eating calming foods and making time to relax.

While the physical activity of the doshas certainly affects our mental state, Ayurveda is specific about subtle, energetic tools for understanding balance in the mind. There are three energies: sattva (the clear essence of the mind) and the two energies that act on it, rajas (restlessness) and tamas (stagnation). The Charaka Samhita considers rajas and tamas to be "doshas of the mind." The three mental energies can be balanced in the same way vata, pitta, and kapha are—by noticing imbalances early on.

Ayurveda is a lifelong exploration and a path to self-realization. Please keep in mind that this chapter is a very basic introduction to these ideas, which have layers of meaning. I wanted to give you just enough information so that we have a simple, common language to illuminate the body/mind connection. It took me ten years of studying Yoga philosophy before I began to feel glimmerings of understanding. I hope to inspire you, with this straightforward cookbook, to enjoy the journey.

CHAPTER 1

Ayurveda: Body, Mind, and Soul

Like other great ancient civilizations, India never separated science from philosophy and religion. Rather, it viewed all knowledge as part of a whole designed to promote human happiness, health, and growth. Philosophy is the love of truth. Science is the discovery of truth through experiment.

Religion is the experience of truth and application of it in daily living. Ayurveda, the science of life, is both systematized knowledge and practical wisdom, an art of healthy living that encompasses all phases of life, body, mind, and spirit. Like all sciences, it includes both a practical and a theoretical aspect. In order to make best use of the practical recommendations that come later in this book, it will help if you understand the essentials of Ayurvedic theory. This first chapter may seem a bit abstract, but please be patient and read it carefully, as it forms the basis of all that is to follow.

The Universe and How We Are Connected

According to Ayurveda, the source of all existence is universal Cosmic Consciousness, which manifests as male and female energy. Purusha, often associated with the male energy, is choiceless, passive, pure awareness. Prakruti, the female energy, is active, choiceful consciousness. Both Purusha and Prakruti are eternal, timeless, and immeasurable. These two energies are present in all living organisms, including every man and woman, as well as inanimate objects.

Purusha is formless and beyond attributes. Unmanifested pure existence, beyond cause and effect, beyond space and time, Purusha takes no active part in creation but remains a silent witness. Prakruti, which has form, color, and attributes, is the divine creative will that dances the dance of creation. Prakruti is the One that becomes many. Purusha is the lover, Prakruti the beloved. Creation of this universe happens through their love. All of nature is the child born from the womb of Prakruti, the Divine Mother.

In the manifestation of nature from Prakruti, the first expression is Mahad (or Mahat), intelligence or cosmic order. (In human beings, it is referred to as Buddhi, intellect.) Next is Ahamkar or ego, the sense of self-identity, the center in our consciousness from which we think, act, and react. Ahamkar expresses itself in three universal qualities:

Sattva is stability, purity, wakefulness, essence, clarity, and light.

Rajas is dynamic movement and causes sensations, feelings, and emotions.

Tamas is the tendency toward inertia, darkness, ignorance, and heaviness. Tamas is responsible for deep sleep and periods of confusion. It also leads to the creation of matter. From the essence of Sattva are born the mind, the five sense faculties and their organs (ears to hear, skin to perceive touch, eyes to see, tongue to taste, nose to smell), and the five motor organs or organs of action: the mouth (for speech), the hands, feet, reproductive organs, and organs of excretion.

Rajas is the active force behind the movement of both the sensory and motor organs.

Tamas gives rise to the five elements, which form the basis of material creation: space (ether), air, fire, water, and earth.

Man, a creation of Cosmic Consciousness, is considered to be a microcosm of the macrocosm that is the universe. Whatever is present in the cosmos, the same is present in human beings. Man is a miniature of nature.

The Five Elements: Building Blocks of Nature

The concept of the five elements is one of the most fundamental in Ayurvedic science. These five elements (space, air, fire, water, and earth) exist in all matter, both organic and inorganic. As man is a microcosm of nature, the five elements also exist within each individual. Our psychological tendencies, as well as our five senses and the various aspects of our body's functioning, are all directly related to the five elements.

According to Ayurveda, the five elements manifest sequentially, beginning with space, from the pure, unified, unmanifested Cosmic Consciousness that is the source of all.

SPACE

Sometimes referred to as "ether," space is empty, light, subtle, all-pervading, omnipresent, and all-enclosing. It is universal, non-moving, and formless. Space is nuclear energy. It appears when the pure unmanifest consciousness begins to vibrate and is associated with sound and the sense of hearing. We need space in order to live, move, grow, and communicate. Spaces in the body include the mouth, nose, gastrointestinal tract, respiratory tract, abdomen, and thorax. Psychologically, space gives freedom, peace, and expansion of consciousness and is responsible for love and compassion as well as feelings of separation, isolation, emptiness, ungroundedness, insecurity, anxiety, and fear.

AIR

Air is dry, light, clear, and mobile. The second manifestation of consciousness, air moves in space. Air is electrical energy—the electron moves because of the air element. It is formless, but it can be perceived by touch, to which it is related. The principle of movement, air expresses itself in the movements of the muscles, the pulsations of the heart, the expansion and contraction of the lungs. Sensory and neural impulses move to and from the brain under the influence of the air principle, which is also responsible for breathing, ingestion, the movement of the intestines, and elimination. The flow of thought, desire, and will are governed by the air principle, which gives us happiness, freshness, joy, and excitation. It is, along with space, also responsible for fear, anxiety, insecurity, and nervousness.

FIRE

Fire is hot, dry, sharp, penetrating, and luminous. When air begins to move, it produces friction, which generates heat or fire. Fire is radiant energy. On the atomic level, the atom radiates heat and light in the form of a quantum wave. Fire is active and changeable. In our solar system, the sun is the source of fire and light. In the body, our biological "fire" in the solar plexus regulates body temperature and metabolism: digestion, absorption, and assimilation. Fire is associated with light and with vision. Fire is intelligence. It is necessary for transformation, attention, comprehension, appreciation, recognition, and understanding. Fire is also responsible for anger, hatred, envy, criticism, ambition, and competitiveness.

WATER

The next manifestation of consciousness, water is fluid, heavy, soft, viscous, cold, dense, and cohesive. It brings molecules together. Water is chemical energy (it is the universal chemical solvent). Water is associated with the sense of taste; without moisture the tongue cannot taste anything. Water exists in the body as plasma, cytoplasm, serum, saliva, nasal secretion, cerebrospinal fluid, urine, and sweat. It is necessary for nutrition and to maintain life; without it, our cells could not survive. Water is contentment, love, and compassion. It creates thirst, edema, and obesity.

EARTH

Earth is heavy, hard, rough, firm, dense, slow-moving, and bulky—the most solid of the five elements. It is neither hot nor cold. Earth is mechanical or physical energy. According to

Ayurveda, it is nothing but crystallized or solidified consciousness. It gives strength, structure, and stamina to the body. All the body's solid structures (bones, cartilage, nails, teeth, hair, skin) are derived from the earth element. Earth is associated with the sense of smell. It promotes forgiveness, support, groundedness, and growth. It also creates attachment, greed, and depression, and its absence produces feelings of ungroundedness.

In our body, the electrical energy of the neuron becomes the physical energy of the movement of muscles, mediated through the neurotransmitter, which is chemical. Indeed, all the five elements are present on every level of our physiology, starting with a single cell. Within the cell, the cell membrane is earth, cellular vacuoles are space, cytoplasm is water, nucleic acid and other chemical components of the cell are fire, and movement of the cell is due to the air principle. Every single cell also has mind, intelligence, and consciousness, through which it manifests selectivity and choice. From all the possible nutrients in its environment, every cell chooses its own food—that choice is intelligence at work.

Both in our outer environment and within us, the proportion and balance of these elements is forever shifting, changing with the seasons, the weather, the time of day, the stage of one's life. For health, and often for sheer survival, we have to continuously accommodate ourselves to these changes, through what we eat, what we wear, where we live, and so on. This is a balancing act, playing elements against each other. We use solid earth to build homes, to protect ourselves against changes in air, heat (fire), and water. We use fire to prepare food (made of water and earth).

The Three Doshas: Vata, Pitta, and Kapha

These five great elements combine into three basic energies or functional principles, which are present, in varying degrees, in everything and everybody. Space (ether) and air constitute vata. Fire and water combine to make up pitta. Water and earth constitute kapha.

In our bodies, these three doshas or humors govern our psychobiological functioning. vata–pitta–kapha are present in every cell, tissue, and organ. When in balance, they create health. When out of balance, they are the cause of disease. These three doshas are responsible for the huge variety of individual differences and preferences, and they influence all we are and all we do, from our choices of food to our modes of relating to others. They govern the biological and psychological processes of our body, mind, and consciousness. They regulate the creation, maintenance, and destruction of bodily tissue, and the elimination of waste products. They also govern our emotions. When in balance, they generate noble qualities such as understanding, compassion, and love.

When their balance is disturbed by stress, improper diet, environmental conditions or other factors, they can give rise to negative emotions such as anger, fear, and greed. In Ayurveda, vata is the bodily air principle. It is the energy of movement. Pitta is the principle of fire, the energy of digestion and metabolism. And kapha is the principle of water, the energy of lubrication and structure.

All people have all of these three doshas, but one of them is usually primary, one secondary, and the third least prominent. Thus, each person has a particular pattern of energy, an individual combination of physical, mental, and emotional characteristics that make up his or her constitution (prakruti). Just as everyone has an individual fingerprint that can be identified by a trained practitioner, so everyone has an energy print—a balance or proportion of vata, pitta, and kapha—that is uniquely his or her own.

Health depends on maintaining this proportion in balance. Balance is the natural order of things; imbalance provokes and reflects disorder. Within our bodies there is a constant interplay between order and disorder, which determines our state of health. Health is order; disease is disorder. The internal environment of the body is ceaselessly reacting to the external environment. Disorder occurs when these two are out of harmony with each other. But since order is inherent within disorder, the wise person learns to be aware of the presence of disorder and sets about to reestablish order.

We will see how the three fundamental doshas combine to create the seven constitutional types of Ayurveda, and you will learn your own body type, the key to making lifestyle choices for self-healing and maximum well-being. For the moment, let us look a little more deeply into the characteristics of these three basic energies of life.

VATA

Vata is the energy of movement. Although it is the air principle, it is not considered the same as actual air in the external environment, but rather as the subtle energy that governs biological movement.

Vata is intimately related to our vital life essence, known as prana. Prana is the pure essence of vata. It is the life-force, the play of intelligence. That flow of intelligence is necessary for communication between two cells, and it maintains the life function of both. On a cosmic level, prana is said to be the attraction between Purusha and Prakruti. As the principle of mobility, vata regulates all activity in the body, both mental and physiological. It is responsible for breathing, the blinking of our eyes, the beating of our hearts, and all movement in the cytoplasm and cell membranes. All the impulses in the vast networks of our nervous system are governed by vata.

When vata is in balance, it promotes creativity and flexibility and evokes feelings of freshness, lightness, happiness, and joy. Out of balance, vata produces fear, nervousness, anxiety, even tremors and spasms. Vata is dry, light, cold, subtle, clear, mobile, and dispersing. We shall soon see how these qualities are expressed in a person with a vata constitution.

PITTA

Pitta is translated as fire, but this is not meant literally. Rather, it is the principle of fire, the energy of heating or metabolism. Pitta governs all the biochemical changes that take place within our bodies, regulating digestion, absorption, assimilation, and body temperature.

From the standpoint of modern biology, pitta comprises the enzymes and amino acids that play a major role in metabolism.

Pitta regulates body temperature through the chemical transformation of food. It promotes appetite and vitality.

Not only food is metabolized by us. Every impression coming in from the outside is also processed or "digested" and made a part of us. Thus pitta (when in balance) promotes intelligence and understanding and is crucial in learning. Out-of-balance pitta may arouse fiery emotions such as frustration, anger, hatred, criticism, and jealousy.

Pitta is hot, sharp, light, oily, liquid, pungent, sour, and spreading. These qualities occur in

various ways in people of pitta constitution.

KAPHA

Kapha combines water and earth. It is the energy that forms the body's structure, the glue that holds the cells together. Kapha also supplies the liquid needed for the life of our cells and bodily systems. It lubricates our joints, moisturizes the skin, helps to heal wounds, and maintains immunity. Kapha provides strength, vigor, and stability.

Psychologically, excess kapha is responsible for the emotions of attachment, greed, lust, and envy. When kapha is in balance it expresses itself in tendencies toward love, calmness, and forgiveness.

The qualities of kapha include heavy, slow, cool, oily, damp, smooth, soft, static, viscous, and sweet.

Kapha individuals display these qualities in various ways. Together, these three doshas govern all the body's metabolic activities. Kapha promotes anabolism, the process of building up the body, the growth and creation of new cells as well as cell repair. Pitta regulates metabolism, which is digestion and absorption. Vata triggers catabolism, the necessary deterioration process in which larger molecules are broken down into smaller ones.

Vata, the principle of movement, moves both pitta and kapha, which are immobile. Thus when vata is out of balance, it influences and disturbs the other doshas. The majority of illnesses have aggravated vata at their source.

The whole of life's journey is divided into three major milestones. From birth to age 16 is the kapha age. From 16 to 50 is the age of pitta, and from 50 to 100 the age of vata. In childhood, kapha and the process of anabolism are predominant, as this is the time of greatest physical growth and the structuring of the body. Kapha disorders, such as lung congestion, cough, colds, and mucus secretions, are common at this time. In adulthood, a time of activity and vitality, pitta is most apparent. Vata and the catabolic processes of deterioration take over in old age, bringing vata disorders such as tremors, emaciation, breathlessness, arthritis, and loss of memory.

The Twenty Qualities: An Important Key to Healing

Now we come to another important aspect of Ayurvedic theory, which will help you to make intelligent choices for self-healing. Ayurveda delineates twenty fundamental qualities, which appear in ten pairs:

The Twenty Basic Attributes or Qualities

Heavy—Light

Oily—Dry

Stable—Mobile

Slimy—Rough

Gross—Subtle

Cold—Hot

Slow—Sharp

Soft—Hard

Dense—Liquid

Cloudy—Clear

These qualities are found both in the world around us and in our bodies. Today's weather may feel light or heavy, and it may be liquid or dry, mobile (windy) or stable, hot or cold, cloudy or clear. Food we eat can partake of any of these qualities. Ice cream, for example, is heavy, oily, cold, soft, and liquid. Our skin may be oily or dry, rough or smooth. Our moods, too, can be heavy or light, cloudy or clear; our thinking may be slow or sharp, our mind quiet and stable or mobile and hyperactive, clear or cloudy.

We are constantly affected by changes in these qualities. Cold, windy, clear, dry weather aggravates vata dosha and may lead to colds and any number of vata ailments such as insomnia, constipation, or arthritis. Hot, humid weather aggravates pitta and may lead to outbreaks of irritation and anger as well as physical complaints like acne, eczema, or skin rashes. Cloudy, gray, humid or rainy weather can aggravate kapha, leading to colds and coughs, depression, lethargy, overeating and oversleeping, and weight gain.

Each of these paired qualities represents the extreme on a continuum. The two qualities in each pair influence or affect one another according to two fundamental principles of Ayurveda:

1. Like increases like.
2. Opposites decrease each other.

These principles are a key to healing with Ayurveda. When an imbalance has manifested, successful treatment requires increasing opposite qualities. For example, if there is too much heat (excess pitta), a cool drink, a swim, or some herbs with cooling properties will greatly help pacify pitta and reduce the heat. A person suffering from too much heat will not be helped by playing tennis in the sun, eating spicy foods, or taking a sauna. Similarly, if you are cold and shivering from exposure to cold windy weather, have a bowl of warm soup, wrap up in a blanket, or take a hot bath. These simple remedies immediately make sense when we hear them because they are so natural.

Ayurvedic physicians have carefully observed nature and located these qualities within all things, both organic and inorganic. Ayurvedic treatment consists to a great extent of identifying a person's disorder in terms of these qualities, and setting right any imbalances.

How is this done? Speaking in very general terms, excessive dryness in the body— constipation, dry skin, emaciation, and so on—is frequently associated with aggravated vata; excessive heat—burning urine, irritated eyes, fever, inflammation, anger, or a critical attitude—with aggravated pitta; and undue heaviness—lethargy, overweight, congestion, and excess mucus—with unbalanced kapha. Whatever the symptoms may be, for selftreatment you need to understand them and then adjust your lifestyle—diet, exercise, and so on—to restore a state of balance and health.

The remedies in this book will help you to do this, but essentially it is your own moment-to-moment awareness and self-observation, your sensitivity to your own constitution and your own unique requirements for health, and perhaps most importantly, your willingness to act on your knowledge, that will make all the difference between poor health and a vital, happy, healthy, long life.

CHAPTER 2

How We Can Stay Healthy

The goal of Ayurveda is to maintain the health of a healthy person and heal the illness of a sick person. But staying well is far easier than curing an illness, especially once an imbalance has progressed through the later stages of the disease process. That is why prevention is so strongly emphasized in Ayurvedic medicine. In this chapter we will consider some of the fundamental principles and approaches recommended by Ayurveda for remaining healthy.

Awareness

The master key to remaining healthy is awareness. If you know your constitution, and you can remain alert to how your mind, body, and emotions respond to the changing conditions in your environment and the numerous facets of your daily life, such as the food you eat, you can make informed choices to maintain good health. The cause is the concealed effect and the effect is the revealed cause, as the seed contains the potential tree and the tree reveals the potency of the seed. To treat the cause is to treat the effect, to prevent it from coming to fruition. If a kapha person always has kapha problems in the spring season, such as hay fever, colds, congestion, sinus headaches, and weight gain, such a person should watch his diet and eliminate kapha-producing food like wheat, watermelon, cucumber, yogurt, cheese, candy, ice cream, and cold drinks. (Ice is not good for a kapha person; it will produce congestive disorders.)

The knowledge of the causes of disease, and the understanding that "like increases like" and "opposites balance," give us all the information we need to maintain or restore our health, simply through conscious attention, moment-to-moment awareness of our behavior. If I am living consciously, I may observe that after I ate yogurt two weeks ago, I felt congested and a cold developed. Then it cleared up and I was okay for a few days. When yogurt comes my way again, the memory will come up and my body will say, "Hey, last time you ate yogurt, you got sick!" If I bring lively awareness and listen to my body, it will tell me, "I don't want yogurt." To listen to the body's wisdom, the body's intelligence, is to be aware, and this is one of the most effective ways to prevent disease.

Developing an awareness of the potential causes of imbalance, and of one's moment-tomoment state of well-being, is the necessary first step to maintaining health. The second step is taking action.

Taking Action to Modify the Cause

You can't control the weather, but you can dress properly, so that cold winds, or rain, or summer's heat will not aggravate the doshas. Changes in the weather are a potential cause of doshic imbalance. Windy, cold, dry weather will aggravate vata dosha; hot, sticky weather is sure to provoke pitta; cold, cloudy, wet weather will increase kapha dosha. Once we have knowledge and understanding, it is time to take action. Put on a hat, a scarf, a warm coat; stay out of direct sunlight. Modify the cause. Potential causes of illness and imbalance are constantly arising, both within us and on the outside. The weather is changing, our surroundings are changing, our thoughts and feelings are changing, and stressful situations are coming and going. In response to these changes, we have to act skillfully. As the Bhagavad Gita says, "Skill in action is called yoga."

I have to be smart enough to know my previous history and to learn from it. When I eat garbanzos, I get a stomachache, so this time I should not eat them. Or if there is nothing to eat except garbanzos, then I can add cumin powder, ghee, and a little mustard seed, and it will be suitable for me to eat. The garbanzos' dry, light vatagenic effect will be modified by the moist, oily ghee and the warming spices.

A substantial part of the Ayurvedic pharmacy is the Ayurvedic art of cooking. Adding specific seasonings changes the property of food and can cause a "forbidden" food, one that might have provoked imbalance, to become acceptable. Some people, for example, are sensitive to potatoes. Potatoes give them gas and little aches and pains in the muscles and around the joints. But if they peel off the skin and sauté the potato with ghee and a little turmeric, mustard seed, cumin powder, and cilantro, it mitigates the vata-provoking property of the potato and the body can then handle it. One can take action to modify the cause; the body's response will be different, and that particular causative factor will not have an adverse effect.

This principle applies equally well to psychological factors. You may know that watching violent movies upsets you and gives you nightmares. The violent imagery disturbs your doshic balance, provoking anxiety and fear. You have observed this happening to you; the next time you are confronted with the "opportunity" to subject yourself to a violent movie, you can just say no.

It keeps coming down to the same central issue: consciousness, awareness, finding out, "What is my role in this situation? What do I know? What can I do?"

Restoring Balance

The first step in staying healthy is developing awareness of the potential causes of disease so you can avoid them or deal with them intelligently. The second step is taking action to modify causes you can't avoid or control (such as the weather). The next step is to restore balance once it begins to be lost. The main method for doing this is to apply the opposite quality or qualities.

If you're cold, have some hot soup or take something warm to drink. If you're agitated or upset (perhaps you watched that violent movie against your better judgment), sit down and do some meditation to calm your mind and emotions. If your pitta has been provoked and you're feeling hot under the collar, take a swim or have some sweet cooling fruit. This principle seems so simple and makes such good sense that it is easy to overlook it in practical daily life. But it is extremely powerful and effective. If you apply it, you will find that you can quickly and effortlessly restore balance to your mind and body.

Techniques for Cleansing and Purification

Now we have to consider still another level of self-healing. What if you haven't taken the opportunity to develop awareness, to modify the cause, or to apply opposite qualities to restore balance, and you have begun to get sick? What to do now? The principle of opposites is almost universally valid and helpful at any stage of disease. But once disease has begun to develop, it will not be sufficient. At this stage it becomes necessary to use techniques for cleansing and purifying your body of excess doshas and accumulated toxins.

As we have seen, when the doshas are aggravated because of poor diet, unhealthy lifestyle, negative emotions, or other factors, they first affect agni (the body's biological fire, which governs digestion and assimilation). When agni becomes weakened or disturbed, food is not properly digested. The undigested, unabsorbed food particles accumulate in the gastrointestinal tract and turn into the toxic, sticky substance called ama. In the third ("spread") stage of the disease process, ama clogs the intestines, overflows through other bodily channels such as the blood vessels, and infiltrates the bodily tissues, causing disease.

Ama is thus the root cause of disease. The presence of ama in the system can be felt as fatigue, or a feeling of heaviness. It may induce constipation, indigestion, gas, and diarrhea, or it may generate bad breath, a bad taste in the mouth, stiffness in the body, or mental confusion. Ama can most easily be detected as a thick coating on the tongue. According to Ayurveda, disease is actually a crisis of ama, in which the body seeks to eliminate the accumulated toxicity. Thus the key to prevention of disease—once ama has begun to build up—is to help the body eliminate the toxins.

To remove ama from the system, Ayurveda employs many internal cleansing programs. One of these, most widely known in the West, is a five-procedure program known as panchakarma ("five actions"). The panchakarma programs used at Ayurvedic treatment centers include prepurification methods to prepare the body to let go of the toxins, followed by the purification methods themselves.

The first preparatory step is internal oleation. The patient is asked to drink a specific, small quantity of ghee (clarified butter) every day for several days. The ghee creates a thin film in the body's channels that lubricates them, allowing the ama lodged in the deep connective tissues to move freely, without sticking to the channels, to the gastrointestinal tract for elimination. Internal oleation is done for three to five days or even longer, depending on the individual circumstances.

This is followed by external oleation in the form of oil massage (snehana) and sweating (swedana). Oil is applied to the entire body with a particular kind of massage that helps the toxins move toward the gastrointestinal tract. The massage also softens both the superficial and deep tissues, helping to relieve stress and to nourish the nervous system. Then the individual is given a steam bath, which further loosens the toxins and increases their movement toward the gastrointestinal tract.

After three to seven days of these procedures, the doshas will have become well "ripened." At this point the physician will determine that the patient is ready to eliminate the aggravated doshas and accumulated ama. One of the five karmas or actions is selected as the most expedient route to eliminate the excess doshas. These procedures may include:

- therapeutic vomiting (vamana) to remove toxins and excess kapha from the stomach;
- purgation or laxative therapy (virechana) to help remove ama and excess pitta from the small intestines, colon, kidneys, stomach, liver, and spleen;
- medicated enema therapy (basti) to help remove excess vata from the colon. Aggravated vata is one of the main etiological factors in the manifestation of diseases. If we can control vata through the use of bastis, we have gone a long way toward eliminating the cause of the vast majority of diseases.
- nasya or nasal administration of medication, in which dry herbal powders or oils such

asghee are inserted into the nose to help remove accumulated doshas in the head, sinus, and throat areas, and to clear up breathing.

- rakta moksha, purification of the blood, which is traditionally done in one of two ways.

Bloodletting, in which a small amount of blood is extracted from a vein, is one method, though it is illegal in the United States and is therefore not available here. The second way is to cleanse the blood using blood-purifying herbs such as burdock. Panchakarma is not the only method used by Ayurveda to remove ama from the body. Depending on the individual's strength and the seriousness of the disease, one of two main approaches will be employed. If the person is weak and debilitated and the disease is strong, the preferred method is palliation and pacification (shamanam), which neutralizes ama through gentler methods of purification, including herbs. If the patient has more strength and energy and the illness is not so complicated or serious, then panchakarma is appropriate.

IMPORTANT NOTE: Panchakarma is a special, powerful procedure requiring guidance from

a properly trained medical staff, not just someone with a modest amount of Ayurvedic training. It is performed individually for each person, with his or her specific constitution and medical condition in mind, and it requires close observation and supervision at every stage, including post-panchakarma support.

A Simple Home Purification

Both for periodic prevention (to reverse any buildup of ama) and to deal with a specific health problem, panchakarma is a highly recommended art of cleansing and detoxification. If you are not near a center where panchakarma is available under the supervision of a trained Ayurvedic physician, you can do an effective purification program at home. Begin your home detoxification program with internal oleation. For three days in a row, take about 2 ounces of warmed, liquefied ghee early in the morning.

For a vata person, take the ghee with a pinch of rock salt.

For a pitta individual, take the 2 ounces of ghee plain. The kapha individual should add to the ghee just a pinch of trikatu (a mixture of equal amounts of ginger, black pepper, and pippali, or Indian long pepper). The ghee provides internal oleation and lubrication, which is necessary so that the ama or toxins begin to come back from the deep tissue to the gastrointestinal tract for elimination. After your three days of internal oleation, it is time for external oleation. For the next five to seven days, apply 7 to 8 ounces of warmed (not hot!) oil to your body from head to toe, rubbing it in well. The best oil for vata types is sesame, which is heavy and warming; pittas should use sunflower oil, which is less heating; kaphas do best with corn oil. You can do this oil massage for fifteen to twenty minutes.

After the oil is well rubbed in and absorbed, take a hot bath or shower. Then wash with some Ayurvedic herbal soap, such as neem. Let some of the oil remain on your skin. The ancient Ayurvedic textbooks recommend rubbing some chickpea flour over the skin to absorb and help remove the oil. This works very well to remove the oil, but it is more suited to a culture in which individuals bathe outdoors. Today, if you use chickpea flour, be aware that oil, flour, and hot water combine into a formidable mass that can easily clog your plumbing. Flushing the drain with extra hot water immediately following your bath can help.

During your home purification, every night at least one hour after supper take ½ to 1 teaspoon of triphala. Add about half a cup of boiling water to the triphala powder, and let it steep ten minutes or until it has cooled down, then drink it. Along with its many healing and nourishing properties, triphala is a mild but effective laxative. It will provide the benefits of a more potent virechana or purgative treatment, but more gently and over a longer span of time. Triphala is safe and can be effectively used for months at a time.

To complete your home panchakarma treatment, on the last three days perform an Ayurvedic medicated enema, or basti, after your hot bath or shower. Use dashamoola tea for the enema. Boil 1 tablespoon of the herbal compound dashamoola in

1 pint of water for five minutes to make a tea. Cool it, strain it, and use the liquid as an enema.

Retain the liquid as long as you comfortably can. And don't worry if little or no liquid comes out. For certain individuals, particularly vata types, the colon may be so dry and dehydrated that the liquid may all be absorbed. This is not harmful in any way.

This snchana (oleation both internal and external with ghee and oil), swedana (sweating using a hot shower or hot bath), and virechana (purgation) using triphala, followed by basti using dashamoola tea, constitute an effective panchakarma that you can easily do on your own at home.

During this entire time it is important to get plenty of rest, and to observe a light diet. From day four to day eight, eat only kitchari (equal amounts of basmati rice and mung dal cooked with cumin, mustard seed, and coriander, with about 2 teaspoons of ghee added to it). Kitchari is a wholesome, nourishing, balanced food that is an excellent protein combination. It is easy to digest and good for all three doshas, and it is also cleansing.

Be your own healer. Do this simple home purification, preferably at the junction between seasons. Take responsibility for your own healing. You will start to experience a great change in your thinking and in your feelings, and you will really fall in love with your life!

Rejuvenation and Rebuilding

The purpose of panchakarma is not just to get well but to purify the body and strengthen it so that future diseases will not occur, and you can enjoy a long life in good health. In this regard the panchakarma purification can be seen as a preliminary to rejuvenation. If you want to dye your shirt, don't color it while it's dirty. Wash it first, then dye it. The washing is the panchakarma detoxification program, and the dyeing is the rejuvenation and revitalization.

Ayurvedic rejuvenatives (rasayanas) bring renewal and longevity to the cells, and when the cells live longer, the person lives longer. Rasayanas give strength, vitality, and longevity, strengthen tone, increase energy, and build immunity. The body's various agnis become more robust, so health becomes more robust. For a vata individual, an excellent rejuvenative tonic is the herb ashwagandha. Take 1 teaspoon of ashwagandha in a cup of hot milk twice a day, morning and evening.

An excellent rejuvenative herb for pittas is shatavari. Take 1 teaspoon twice a day in a cup of warm milk. Kaphas can use punarnava, 1 teaspoon twice a day, but in a cup of warm water.

You can also use various herbal mixtures designed to tonify the system, such as the traditional recipe chyavanprash.

Three Cautions About Home Panchakarma

1. Panchakarma, even in this gentle home program, has a powerful effect and should be done only by individuals of sufficient strength. If you are anemic, or feel weak and debilitated, even this home procedure is not for you.

2. Do not do panchakarma in a clinic, or even this home purification, if you are pregnant.

3. One result of panchakarma, even in this mild home version, is that the deep connective tissue may start releasing unresolved past emotions, such as grief, sadness, fear, or anger along with the built-up ama and excess doshas. If this happens, make yourself some Tranquillity Tea, and meditate, using whatever

method you have learned or the Empty Bowl meditation described. The releasing of emotions may happen weeks or even several months after you finish your home panchakarma. To make your rejuvenation more effective, after completing your panchakarma purification program, set some time aside to build up your strength. Whether you take a weekend, a week, a month, or even more, use the time as a purposeful period of rest, relaxation, and rebuilding of body, mind, and spirit. Here are a few suggestions:

Get plenty of rest.

Observe celibacy so that you don't waste your vital energy.

Eat carefully, according to the guidelines for your constitution.

Meditate and do yoga postures regularly.

Self-Esteem

Self-esteem is at the core of healing. Because of the connectedness of mind and body, our sense of self-esteem is our cells' sense of self-esteem. This is because, according to Ayurveda, every cell is a center of intelligence and awareness. Every cell carries the sense of self for its own survival. It is the sense of self in the cell that maintains the size and shape of the cell.

Self-esteem, self-confidence, and self-respect promote cellular intelligence, which is necessary for proper cell function and immunity. Modern science is just now acknowledging the importance of the mind-body connection, but knowledge of it has been part of Ayurveda for five thousand years. Our sense of self, our attitudes and understandings, our feelings, are all psychobiological events. Self-esteem is one such event, one that is strengthening to our cells and to all aspects of our bodies. A lack of self-confidence and self-love is detrimental.

Cancer is an example of this lack. Cancer cells have lost their intelligence and grow separate from the body. They are irregular and robust and have an isolated, selfish sense of self which is in conflict with the life of normal, healthy cells. When cancer occurs, it's as if a war is going on between the cancerous cells and the healthy cells. If the healthy cells are strong enough in self-esteem, they can conquer and kill the cancer cells. But if we do not have enough self-esteem and self-respect, then the cancer cells will win and will conquer the healthy cells.

Thus self-esteem is important for maintaining immunity. If you love yourself as you are, you will develop confidence, and that will heal disease. That is why cellular immunity, or natural resistance, depends upon self-esteem.

Ayurvedic Lifestyle: The Ultimate Preventive Medicine

How you live your daily life is the key factor in determining your health and your quality of experience. It is also the factor over which you have the most control. You can't control the weather or your genetic makeup, but what you do every day either builds up your health, vitality, and resistance to disease, or wears you down. Your moment-tomoment choices—what to eat, how much to eat, how to respond to others, whether to exercise or not, how late to stay up at night, and so on—play a major role in your mental and physical health.

But how do you create your lifestyle, the rhythms of your daily living? Is it just pure habit, based on how your parents lived and how you grew up? Should the time you wake up be dictated by when you need to get to work, and should what you eat be determined by what's available at the fast-food shops? If you decide to take control of your lifestyle and structure new, healthier habits, what principles will guide you?

According to Ayurveda, you couldn't do better than to strive to live your life in harmony with Mother Nature.

In Tune with Nature

Ayurveda flourished in a civilization vastly different from life today, a world in which human life was intimately intertwined with the life of nature. The great rhythms and forces of nature—the alternation of day and night, the rhythmic cycle of seasons—all affect us, as do the inevitable seasons and cycles of human life, birth and growth, aging and death. Through the plants we eat for food, the water we drink, and the air we breathe in common with all beings, we are inextricably one with nature.

The sages of settled mind who unfolded the wisdom of Ayurveda saw this, and they saw that the master key to good health is to get ourselves into harmony with nature. Thus the ideal Ayurvedic daily routine that follows is, as you will see, based on patterns of nature.

Being in tune with nature also means being in tune with your nature, your constitution or prakruti (which means nature). It means being true to your own nature, to how you are built, mentally and emotionally as well as physically. It means that your food and exercise requirements, how much you need to sleep, how much sexual activity is healthy for you, what kind of climate is beneficial, all revolve around your doshic makeup, your individual nature.

Living in accordance with nature and natural law means continually balancing our inner ecology by adjusting to our ever-changing environment.

Ayurvedic Daily Routine

A daily routine is essential for maintaining good health and for transforming our body, mind, and consciousness to a higher level of functioning. A regulated daily routine puts us in harmony with nature's rhythms. It establishes balance in our constitution and helps to regularize our biological clock. It indirectly aids in digestion, absorption, and assimilation of food, and it generates self-esteem, discipline, peace, happiness, and long life. Waking up too early or too late, undisciplined eating, staying up too late, job stress, and untimely bowel movements are a few habits that can unsettle us. Regularity in sleeping, waking, eating, and eliminating, indeed following a regular daily routine, brings discipline to life and helps maintain the integrity of the doshas.

Our body is a clock. Or rather, it is several clocks at once. According to Ayurveda, every organ has a definite time of maximum functioning. Morning time is the lung time. Midday is stomach time, when we feel hungry. Afternoon is liver time, and late afternoon is when the colon and kidneys operate at their peak.

This biological clock works in conjunction with the doshic clock. Morning and evening (dawn and dusk) are the times when the influence of vata is greatest. In the early morning, from about 2 A.M. to sunrise, vata creates movement and people awaken and tend to excrete waste. Again in the late afternoon, from about 2 P.M. until sunset, the influence of vata makes one feel light and active.

Early morning and evening are kapha times. From sunrise until about 10 A.M., kapha makes one feel fresh but a little heavy. Then again in the evening, from about 6 P.M. until around 10, kapha ushers in a period of cooling air, inertia, and declining energy.

Midday and midnight are pitta times. At midmorning, kapha slowly merges into pitta, and by noon one feels hungry and ready for lunch. Again from 10 P.M. until around 2 A.M., pitta is at its peak, and food is digested.

Thus there is a daily cycle of vata–pitta–kapha:

6 A.M.–10 A.M. = kapha
10 A.M.–2 P.M. = pitta
2 P.M.–6 P.M. = vata
6 P.M.–10 P.M. = kapha
10 P.M.–2 A.M. = pitta
2 A.M.–6 A.M. = vata

So there is a doshic clock (when a particular dosha is operating at its peak) and a biological clock (when a particular organ is operating at its peak). Based on these clocks, the Ayurvedic sages developed the dinacharya, or daily routine. This daily routine is the art of bringing harmony between the biological and doshic clocks and chronological time. Here are its most salient features:

WAKE UP EARLY

It is beneficial to wake up before the sun rises. At this time of the morning, pure qualities are lively in nature, which can bring freshness to the doors of perception and peace of mind.

Ideally, vata people should get up at about 6 A.M., pitta people by 5:30, and kapha people by 4:30. This is the ideal: do the best you can. If you can wake up at 5:30, it will be very good.

Right after awakening, look at your hands for a few moments, then gently move them over your face, neck, and chest down to your waist. This will bring more alertness.

SAY A PRAYER

It is good to start the day by remembering the Divine Reality that is our life. You may do this in your own way, as your religion or personal experience dictates. Or you may use this simple prayer:

Dear God, you are inside of me

Within my very breath

Within each bird, each mighty mountain.

Your sweet touch reaches everything

and I am well protected.

Thank you God

for this beautiful day before me.

May joy, love, peace, and compassion

be part of my life

and all those around me on this day.

I am healing and I am healed.

WASH YOUR FACE, MOUTH, AND EYES

Splash your face with cold water a couple of times. Swish and rinse out your mouth. Then wash your eyes with cool water, and massage the eyelids by gently rubbing them. Blink your eyes seven times, and then rotate your eyes in all directions: side to side, up and down, diagonally, clockwise, and counterclockwise. All this will help you feel alert and fresh.

DRINK A GLASS OF WATER

Drink a glass of room-temperature water, preferably from a pure copper cup or tumbler. (Fill the cup the night before and let it sit overnight.) If the water is too cold, it may provoke kapha disorders such as colds, coughs, and sore throat. For kapha and vata individuals, it is actually better to drink hot water, but for a pitta person, lukewarm is best. This water will not be absorbed but will wash the gastrointestinal tract and flush the kidneys. It also stimulates peristalsis in the intestines, stimulates the descending colon and ileocecal valve, and helps with having a good bowel movement.

It is not a good idea to start the day with coffee or black tea. These drain kidney energy, overstimulate the adrenals, and promote constipation. They are also habit-forming.

EVACUATION

Sit (or better, squat) on the toilet, and have a bowel movement. Even if you don't have the urge, sit for a few minutes, without forcing. If you do this every day, following your glass of warm water, the habit will develop.

After evacuation, wash the anal orifice with warm water, then wash your hands with a gentle soap.

CLEAN YOUR TEETH AND TONGUE

Use a soft toothbrush for your teeth, and an herbal powder made of astringent, pungent, and bitter herbs. Scrape your tongue every morning. This is an important part of daily hygiene, from which you can learn a lot about your health and habits. Note how coated your tongue is, and how your breath smells. If you get the smell of last night's pizza, that means the food is not yet thoroughly digested. If there is a lot of coating on the tongue, that means there is much ama or toxicity in the system. Perhaps you ate too late, or your dinner was hard to digest.

If there is ama on the tongue and a bad smell on the breath, don't eat breakfast. Eating breakfast is not good if you have not digested last night's dinner.

You can see that this daily regimen brings more awareness. By following this routine, you come in contact with your body and observe the functioning of your system. You know exactly what is happening. This knowledge gives you the power to create better health by altering your behavior.

To scrape your tongue, use a stainless-steel tongue scraper. You can also use a spoon. Gently scrape from the back or base of the tongue forward, until you have scraped the whole surface (seven to fourteen strokes). In addition to removing bacteria from the tongue, scraping sends an indirect message to all the internal organs and stimulates gastric fire and digestive enzymes.

GARGLE

To strengthen the teeth, gums, and jaw, to improve the voice and remove wrinkles from the cheeks, gargle twice a day with warm sesame oil. Also, hold the oil in your mouth and swish it around vigorously. Then spit it out and gently massage the gums with your index finger.

NOSE DROPS (NASYA)

Now put 3 to 5 drops of warm ghee, brahmi ghee, or sesame oil into each nostril. This helps to clean the sinuses and also improves voice, vision, and mental clarity. In dry climates, and during cold winters when the house is heated with dry air, nose drops help to keep the nostrils lubricated. The nose is the doorway to the brain. Use of nose drops nourishes prana and enlivens consciousness and intelligence.

OIL MASSAGE

Take 4 or 5 ounces of warm (not hot) oil, and rub it all over your head and body. Gently massaging the scalp with oil can bring happiness into your day, as well as help prevent headaches and slow balding and graying of your hair. If you oil your body again before going to bed, it will help induce sound sleep.

Oil massage improves circulation, calms the mind, and reduces excess vata. The skin of the entire body becomes soft, smooth, and brightened.

Best Oils by Body Type

For Ayurvedic oil massage, use one of the following oils, according to your constitutional type:

Vata = sesame oil

Pitta = sunflower oil

Kapha = corn oil

BATHING

Following your oil massage, take a bath or shower. Bathing is cleansing and refreshing. It removes fatigue, brings energy and alertness, and promotes long life. Bathing every day brings holiness into your life.

EXERCISE

Everyone should do some exercise every day. A walk in the fresh early-morning air and some yoga stretching are good enough for many people; some additional aerobic exercise may also be beneficial, depending on your prakruti.

Kapha individuals, with their stronger, heavier physiques, can do the most strenuous exercise, and they benefit from it. Jogging, bicycling, tennis, aerobics, hiking, and mountain climbing are great for kaphas (though they don't like such vigorous exercise!). Pittas do well with a moderate amount (swimming is especially helpful for cooling pitta), while vata individuals do best with quieter exercises like walking, easy swimming, or yoga asanas.

As a general rule, Ayurveda recommends exercising up to one half of one's capacity. A good gauge is to exercise until sweat forms on the forehead, under the arms, and along the spinal column. Straining is absolutely not recommended. Yoga stretching is recommended for all body types. Postures particularly beneficial for vata individuals include the Sun Salutation (twelve cycles, done slowly). The most important seat of vata in the body is in the pelvic cavity, and any exercise that stretches the pelvic muscles helps to calm vata. These include the Forward Bend, Backward Bend, Spinal Twist, Shoulder Stand, Plow, Camel, Cobra, Locust, Cat, and Cow poses, and Leg Lifts. The Headstand, Half Wheel, and Yoga Mudra are also beneficial.

The major seat of pitta is the solar plexus, so exercises that stretch the muscles around the solar plexus are especially beneficial for individuals with a pitta prakruti and will help to pacify pitta. These include the Fish, Boat, Camel, Locust, and Bow poses. Pittas should also do the Moon Salutation (sixteen cycles, moderately fast). Avoid the Headstand, Shoulder Stand, Plow, and other inverted poses.

The important seat of kapha is in the chest. Exercises that stretch the pulmonary cavity and increase circulation in the chest are effective for kaphas and will help relieve and prevent bronchial congestion, cough, and other kapha illnesses. Beneficial postures include the Sun Salutation (twelve cycles, done rapidly) and the Shoulder Stand, Plow, Locust, Bridge, Peacock, Palm Tree, and Lion postures.

PRANAYAMA

After finishing your exercises, sit quietly and do some deep breathing: twelve Alternate Nostril breaths for vata; sixteen Cooling (shitali) breaths for pitta; one hundred Breath of Fire (bhastrika) breaths for kapha.

MEDITATION

End your pranayama by going right into your meditation. Whatever system or technique of meditation you do, do it now. If you don't presently do any meditation practice, try the Empty Bowl meditation. You will find that meditation brings peace and balance into your life.

BREAKFAST

Now it is time for you to enjoy your breakfast! Your meal should be fairly light in the hot months, and more substantial in cold weather. Vata and pitta persons should eat some breakfast; kaphas are usually better off if they don't eat, since eating during kapha time will increase kapha in the body. Follow the dietary guidelines for the three doshas.

OFF TO WORK

After breakfast go to work or to your studies if you are a student. While walking to work (or to and from your car, the train, or the bus), be aware of every step. Carry your meditative mind with you. When you look at your boss or colleague, at the same time look inside. Then your work will become a meditation. You will find yourself looking at others with compassion and greater awareness.

It is better not to drink tea or coffee at work. If you are thirsty, have some warm water or some fruit juice if you prefer.

LUNCHTIME

By around noon you will become quite hungry. Have a bowl of soup and some salad, or some rice and vegetables, following the guidelines for your constitution. And don't drink too much during your meal. Take a cup of water (preferably warm but definitely not iced), and just take a sip between two mouthfuls of food. Drinking a little water improves digestion. One can drink a cup of water an hour before lunch or an hour after lunch, but not immediately afterward, as that slows down digestion and creates ama.

SIT STRAIGHT, WALK STRAIGHT

Maintain your vertebral column straight. When you keep the backbone straight, energy flows upward and you maintain your awareness. It is difficult to be aware when the spine is crunched.

TAKE A WALK

When you've finished your job for the day, go home and take a walk, alone, silently, in the woods, in the park, or on the bank of the river. Listen to the water, the birds, the rustle of leaves, the barking of a dog. In that listening, the meditative mind is regained. In this way, every day becomes heavenly. Every day becomes a celebration, something new. That's why the routine is most important. The discipline of the routine leaves room for awareness, openness, and freshness.

SUPPER TIME

At around six o'clock have your supper. If you like to cook, you can cook according to the Ayurvedic Cookbook for Self-Healing that I have written with my wife, Usha Lad. Don't watch television while eating. Pay attention to the food. Eating food with attention becomes meditation. And when you are eating with awareness, you will not eat too much; you'll eat just a sufficient amount. It is better to eat when the sun is up. Eating late at night will change the body chemistry, sleep will be disturbed, and you will not feel rested in the morning. If you eat supper around 6, by 9 the stomach will be empty and you will sleep soundly.

AFTER DINNER

Sing songs while you wash the dishes. Be happy. Keep smiling. About an hour after dinner, if you are taking triphala (an herbal compound that is both strengthening and purifying), take ½ teaspoon with some warm water. Then if you like, you can watch TV, perhaps some news. You should know what's happening in this world of ours. Or you can read a magazine or a book.

BEFORE GOING TO BED

Before you go to bed, some spiritual reading is important, even if only for a few minutes. And don't forget to drink a cup of hot milk, with a little ginger, cardamom, and turmeric. Drinking milk at bedtime helps to induce sound sleep. According to Ayurveda, that milk also nourishes shukra dhatu, the body's highly refined reproductive tissue.

Rubbing a little oil on the soles of your feet and on the scalp is also soothing and promotes restful sleep.

Finally, before you go to bed, do a few minutes of meditation. Sit quietly and watch your breath. In the pauses between breaths, you'll meet with nothingness, and nothingness is energy and intelligence. Allow that intelligence to deal with your problems. In this way, you'll begin and end your day with meditation, and meditation will stay with you even during deep sleep.

BEDTIME

It is recommended that vatas go to bed by 10 P.M. and sleep on their left side. Pittas should sleep on the right side, retiring between 10 and 11 P.M. The best bedtime for kapha individuals is between 11 and midnight; they should sleep on their left side.

Kapha individuals generally like to sleep about nine hours, and they feel it is good for them. But this is an illusion. Sleeping this long will slow down their metabolism, and they will put on weight and become chubby. The best schedule for them is to stay up until about 11 P.M. or midnight, then to wake up early, around 4:30 or 5:00 A.M. and go out for a walk.

That shorter sleep will help to induce a light quality in their body, and they will start losing weight.

SEX

Ayurveda has some definite suggestions about the proper role of sex in our lives. Sex is a tremendous creative force, and through sex people share their love and compassion and can

derive great pleasure.

Sex is also correlated with constitutional type. The recommended frequency of sexual activity is quite different for the different types. Kaphas, with their strong constitutions, can make love two to three times a week, whereas the suggestion for vatas is once or at most twice a month. Pitta individuals are in the middle; every two weeks is recommended for them.

Too-frequent lovemaking reduces ojas, the body's vital energy, and leaves the person weak and open to diseases. It also aggravates vata dosha.

To restore strength and replenish ojas, after each time you make love a massage is helpful, as are nourishing drinks such as almond milk. The best time for lovemaking is between 10 and 11 P.M. Sex in the morning or in the daytime is not recommended.

This entire daily routine is very important.

I set more store by a good regimen that maintains my humors in balance and procures me a sound sleep. Drink hot when it freezes, drink cool in the dog days; in everything, neither too much nor too little; digest, sleep, have pleasure, and snap your fingers at the rest of it.

Seasonal Routines

The seasons, like the times of day, are characterized by cycles of vata, pitta, and kapha. Maintaining good health during all four seasons requires living in harmony with these natural cycles, continually adjusting to the changes in the outer environment through the food we choose to eat, the type and amount of exercise we do, the clothes we wear, and so on. The suggestions in this section will help you be at your best all year round.

Please remember that you cannot determine the seasons just by dates on the calendar. Ayurveda is a system of natural medicine, which means that you have to see what is happening in nature! In different geographic areas the seasons come at different times and have varied characteristics. In addition, in just one day there may be four seasons: sunshine and singing birds creating a springlike air in the morning; warm summery breezes at midday; gusts of cool, dry autumnal wind in the afternoon; cold, cloudy, wintry weather after dark. So look at nature as it is, and apply the appropriate principles and practices.

GUIDELINES FOR SUMMER

Summer is hot, bright, and sharp, the season of pitta. Thus the main recommendation for everyone, especially for individuals whose prakruti is primarily pitta, is to keep cool and not allow pitta dosha to become aggravated.

- In the morning, as part of your daily routine, rub 5 to 6 ounces of coconut oil or sunflower oil on your body before bathing. Coconut oil is calming, cooling, and soothing to the skin.

- Wear cotton or silk clothing; it is cooling, light, and allows the skin to breathe. Loosefitting clothes are best; they permit the air to pass through and cool the body.
- The best colors to wear in hot weather are white, gray, blue, purple, and green. Avoid red, orange, dark yellow, and black, which absorb and retain heat and will aggravate pitta.
- Follow the pitta-pacifying diet from the food guidelines. Good fruits for summer include apples, pears, melons, plums, and prunes. Watermelon and lime juice are also good in summer. Try steamed asparagus, broccoli, brussels sprouts, cucumber raita, and basmati rice. Kitchari made of basmati rice and mung dal, with a little ghee and grated coconut, makes a delicious light meal. Avoid

sour fruits, citrus fruits, and even beets and carrots, which are all heating. Garlic, onion, chili, tomato, sour cream, and salted cheeses are also not recommended. You can eat more salads in summer than at any other time, as they are cooling, but they are best eaten for lunch. If you eat meat, you can have some light meat—chicken, turkey, or shrimp—once a week. Avoid dark meats, which are heating.

- Don't drink hot water or hot drinks in the summer. Room-temperature or cool drinks are best. Ice and iced drinks, however, inhibit digestion and create toxins (ama) in the body; it is best never to drink them.

- A refreshing drink is cool lassi. Mix 1 part yogurt with 4 parts water, and blend 2 or 3 minutes until creamy. You can add ¼ teaspoon roasted cumin seed before blending, or for a sweet-flavored drink, add 2 tablespoons Sucanat or other sweetener and 1 drop of rose water. The juice of ¼ lime in a cup of cool water with a pinch of cumin powder is also refreshing.

- Working in a hot kitchen provokes pitta. If you cook, cook in the early morning or in the evening. If someone cooks three days in a row, on the fourth day you should treat that person to dinner in a restaurant. This will avoid conflicts in the relationship.
- If you customarily drink alcoholic beverages, avoid whiskey, brandy, rum, and red wine, which are heating. Some cool beer during hot days will be all right.
- This is a season of generalized low energy. Thus it is all right to take a short nap in the daytime.
- If you have to work outside, wear a wide-brimmed hat.

- Wear sunglasses outdoors during the brightest part of the day. Lenses should be smoky gray or green, not red or yellow and especially not blue or purple, which will damage the eyes.
- If you can, work indoors. Have some air conditioning in your car and in your room or office.
- Never lie in the sun in summer. If the weather is very hot, don't wear shorts or short sleeves, but wear loose-fitting clothing to protect your skin. No person having multiple moles should lie in the sun; it may provoke extreme pitta aggravation and lead to skin cancer.
- If you feel really hot, take a swim in a cool lake or pool, then drink a little lime juice in water.
- Avoid strenuous exercise. If you are accustomed to running or other vigorous

aerobic exercise, do it early in the morning at the coolest part of the day.

- Do some mild yoga exercises and quiet meditation twice a day. Good postures for summer include the Fish, Camel, Boat, Cobra, Cow, and Palm Tree poses. Pitta individuals should not do inverted poses such as Headstand and Shoulder Stand, which can be pittaprovoking.

  Also, do the Moon Salutation.

- Perform shitali pranayama, a cooling breathing exercise described.
- Certain jewelry and gems will help cool pitta. These include a necklace of sandalwood beads, a jade or pearl necklace, amethyst crystals, moonstone, malachite crystals, and any silver jewelry.
- In the evening, after dinner, go for a walk in the moonlight. Dress in white clothes, with

white flowers in your hair or a garland of white flowers around your neck.

- You can go to bed a little later on summer nights, around 11 P.M. or midnight. Rub some coconut oil on your scalp and the soles of your feet for a cooling effect before going to sleep. Sleep on your right side.
- Sandalwood, jasmine, and khus oils are cooling and are good fragrances to wear in the summer. Also, place a few drops of sandalwood oil on your pillow, and you will be sleeping with sandalwood perfume all night.
- Sex should be minimized in the summer, as it is heating and will provoke pitta. If you want to have sex, do it between 9 and 10 P.M., when it is cooler but not yet pitta time.

During the summer, the sun evaporates the moisture of the earth and therefore induces hot, dry and sharp qualities in the atmosphere, resulting in pitta aggravation. In summer sweet, cold, liquid, and fatty food and drinks are beneficial.

One should avoid or minimize excessive exercise and sex, alcohol, and diets which are salty, sour, pungent, or hot. In summer time one should enjoy forests, gardens, flowers, and cool water. During the night one should sleep on the open airy roof of the house, which is cooled by the rays of the moon.

GUIDELINES FOR FALL

Autumn is dry, light, cold, windy, rough, and empty (trees drop their leaves). All these qualities provoke vata dosha. So naturally the guidelines for autumn revolve around pacifying vata.

- If you can, wake up early, around 5 A.M., when the air is calm and the birds are not yet out of bed. There is an extraordinary silence and peace at this time of day.

- Good yoga asanas for the autumn season include the Lotus pose, Forward Bend, Backward Bend, Vajrasana (Sitting on the Heels), Spinal Twist, Camel, Cobra, Cow, and Cat. Shoulder Stand and Headstand are all right in moderation. Also do the Sun Salutation a minimum of twelve cycles. As a maximum, you can do as many Sun Salutations as your age, but you have to build up to this through regular daily practice. Finish your yoga session with savasana, the relaxation pose.

- Gentle Alternate Nostril pranayama is good following yoga postures. Then meditate for at least ten to fifteen minutes.

- Every morning before your bath or shower, rub 6 to 9 ounces of warm sesame oil all over your body, from head to toe. Sesame oil is warming and heavy and will help to balance vata. Then take a nice warm shower. Leave a little of the oil on your skin.

- Good fall colors for pacifying vata are red, yellow, and orange. White is also helpful.
- After your yoga, meditation, and bath, have some breakfast. Try oatmeal, cream of rice, cream of wheat, tapioca, or any grain that will help to settle vata. For lunch and supper, tortillas, chapatis, basmati rice, mung dal kitchari, and steamed vegetables are all good fall foods to balance vata. Salads are not recommended. Mushy, soft soups and stews are good, and be sure to use some ghee.
- Don't drink black tea or coffee after dinner. Try some herbal tea, such as cumincoriander- fennel tea (equal proportions), or ginger-cinnamon-clove tea.

- Fasting is not good during the autumn season. It generates too much lightness and emptiness, which provoke vata.
- Be sure to keep warm. Dress warmly enough both indoors and out. On a windy, gusty day, cover your head and ears.
- Very active, vigorous exercise should be avoided, especially by individuals with a vata constitution.
- A short afternoon nap is acceptable for vatas.
- Try to be in bed by 10 P.M.
- Drinking a cup of warm milk at bedtime is good in the autumn season. It induces sound, natural sleep. Heat the milk until it begins to boil and rise up, then let it cool enough to drink comfortably. You might add a pinch each of ginger and cardamom and a small pinch of nutmeg. These herbs are warming and soothing and will help both with digesting the milk and with relaxation.

- At the junction between summer and fall, a panchakarma treatment will help remove excess vata from the system. If you can't go to an Ayurvedic clinic, try the home purification treatment outlined. A crucial component of this treatment should be the basti or medicated enema, as follows:

1. Boil 2 tablespoons of dashamoola powder in 1 pint of water for 5 minutes.
2. Strain out the herbs, and to the liquid add ½ cup warm sesame oil.
3. When this mixture has cooled to a comfortable temperature, use it for the enema. Try to retain it for 30 minutes.
4. After half an hour or after a good bowel movement, add another ½ cup warm sesame oil to the rectum. Try to retain this oil for at least 10 minutes.

- This procedure will lubricate the colon, calm vata, and remove stress from the lower back and neck areas. You can do this basti once a week during the autumn season to keep vata in check.

- During this season, take particular care to avoid loud noise, loud music (such as rock), fast driving, and too much sexual activity. Avoid cold drafts and cold winds. These all aggravate vata.
- Excellent herbs for pacifying vata dosha in the autumn are dashamoola (actually a formula consisting of ten herbs), ashwagandha, bala, and vidari.

GUIDELINES FOR WINTER

In winter, the sky is cloudy, the weather is cold, damp, and heavy, and life in the cities moves slowly; it is generally a season of kapha. A kapha-pacifying regimen should be dopted, especially by kapha individuals. However, certain vata-provoking qualities, such as dry, cold, windy, and clear, are sometimes prominent on winter days, so vata individuals need to keep this in mind.

- In winter there is no need to get up early. The 5:00 rising time suggested for summer and autumn is not necessary now. Unless you have to get up earlier to go to work, you can get up around 7 A.M.
- After brushing your teeth and scraping your tongue, do some yoga asanas, including the Sun Salutation. Beneficial postures for winter season include the Fish, Locust, Boat, Bow, Lion, and Camel poses, Shoulder Stand and Headstand.

These postures help to open the chest, stretch the throat, drain the sinuses, and relieve congestion of the chest.

- Follow your yoga postures with some breathing exercises. Bhastrika (Breath of Fire) will cleanse kapha dosha. Follow this with a few minutes of Right Nostril breathing, which promotes circulation and heat.

- Winter is a season of kapha. So, like slow and steady kapha, don't be in a rush. Be sure to follow your breathing exercises with some quiet meditation.
- After meditation apply some warm sesame oil to your entire body, then take a hot shower. Sesame oil, which is warming, is beneficial for all constitutional types in the winter.
- For a good winter breakfast, have some oatmeal, cornmeal, barley soup, tapioca, kitchari, or poha (cooked rice flakes). About an hour later, drink tea made of these herbs:

dry ginger ½ teaspoon

cinnamon ½ teaspoon

clove a pinch

Boil these herbs in a cup of hot water for five minutes, and drink the tea. It will increase heat and pitta, improve circulation, and eliminate mucus from the system. However, if you have an ulcer, don't drink this tea; it will be too heating.

- Wear bright warming colors such as red and orange.
- Always wear a hat outdoors in winter. More than 60 percent of the body's heat is lost through the head. Also cover your neck and ears.
- For lunch, eat kapha-soothing food but not food that is vata-aggravating. Whole-wheat bread, steamed vegetables, and hot mushy soup with much ghee and some crunchy croutons would be just right.
- If you like to eat meat, Ayurveda says that winter is the time to eat it, because agni (digestive fire) is strong. Chicken and turkey are good choices.

- Although a nap may be acceptable in summer and autumn (especially for pitta and vata individuals, respectively), sleeping in the daytime is not recommended during winter because it will increase kapha, slow down metabolism, and reduce the gastric fire.
- Ayurveda recommends drinking a little dry red wine—a few ounces at most—in the winter to improve digestion and circulation. Draksha (Ayurvedic herbal wine) is a good choice. Take 4 teaspoons of draksha with an equal amount of water before or after dinner.
- The winter season, when the sky is covered by clouds and it is gray outdoors, is conducive to loneliness and depression. Following the kapha-pacifying routine will definitely help. If possible, don't be away from your wife, husband, boyfriend, or girlfriend in the winter. When it is cold outside and inside there is no one to sleep with, you will

definitely feel lonely. When you have your companion in the winter, you feel great!

- At the end of the day, rub a small amount of sesame oil on your scalp and on the soles of your feet.
- According to Ayurvedic tradition, winter is the season in which you can have sex more often.
- The best herbs for winter are pippali, licorice, ginger, punarnava, black pepper, and kutki.

You can also use the herbal tonic chyavanprash.

- Some light fasting, for a day or two, is all right if your digestive fire is strong. You can drink some apple juice or pomegranate juice during your fast if you like.
- At the junction between autumn and winter, individuals who tend to get kapha problems in winter (colds, coughs, flu, sinus congestion, and the like) should receive panchakarma at an Ayurvedic clinic, under the care of an

Ayurvedic physician, to remove excess kapha dosha. This will help give you a problem-free winter.

GUIDELINES FOR SPRING

Spring is the king of the seasons. In the Bhagavad Gita Lord Krishna reveals his predominant attributes in the eleventh chapter: "I am the Soul in the body, the Mind in the senses, the Eagle among birds, the Lion among animals. Among all the trees I am the sacred Bodhi tree, and of the seasons, I am Spring." In spring Mother Earth wakes up and causes sprouting; energy moves up; everything is blooming and flowering, full of colors and greenery. People feel energetic and love to go outdoors. It is the season of celebration.

The qualities of spring are warm, moist, gentle, and unctuous. Due to the warmth, the accumulated snow and ice of winter begin to melt. Similarly, accumulated kapha in the body starts liquefying and running. That is why so many people get spring colds. In addition, as flowers shed their pollen, fragrance, and perfume, making vata and pitta people happy, many kapha individuals get hay fever and allergies.

As early winter carries some of the qualities of fall, so early spring is much like winter, and many of the recommendations are the same. For example, panchakarma is highly recommended, to clear the system of accumulated kapha dosha and help prevent allergies, hay fever, colds, and sinus congestion.

- Good herbs for spring include ginger, black pepper, pippali, and a tea made of cumin, coriander, and fennel in equal proportions. Sitopaladi, punarnava, and sudarshan are also beneficial.

- Strictly avoid heavy, oily food. Also, it is better not to eat sour, sweet, and salty foods, as they provoke kapha. Stay away from dairy products, especially in the morning. Avoid ice cream and cold drinks, which are especially kaphagenic.

- Favor bitter, pungent, and astringent foods. All legumes, such as yellow split peas, red lentils, and garbanzo and pinto beans, are recommended. Radishes, spinach, okra, onions, and garlic can be used, along with hot spices such as ginger, black pepper, cayenne pepper, and chili pepper. (But don't overdo these hot spices if your constitution is predominantly vata or especially if it is pitta.) After each meal, drink some tea made from ginger, black pepper, and cinnamon.

- Use less ghee and fewer dairy products, and use more honey, which is heating. A cup of hot water with a teaspoon of honey helps balance kapha during the spring season. (But never cook honey; it clogs the subtle channels and acts as a toxin in the system.) You can end your meal with a cup of freshly made lassi.

- For those who eat meat, chicken, turkey, rabbit, and venison are permissible; seafood, crab, lobster, and duck are not recommended during spring season.
- This is a good season to observe a juice fast of apple, pomegranate, or berry juice.
- Wake up early, and go for a morning walk. Also, do the Sun Salutation and kaphareducing

yoga postures, such as the Fish, Boat, Bow, Locust, Lion, and Camel poses, and the Headstand and/or Shoulder Stand. Bhastrika and Right Nostril breathing are also helpful

- Sleeping in the daytime aggravates kapha; hence it is not recommended during this season.

As spring advances and the weather heats up, you will want to change from a kaphapacifying

regimen to the pitta-pacifying guidelines suggested for summer. In fact, as the weather alternates between cold and hot, you will need to be alert day-to-day and use your common sense to remain in balance.

Ayurvedic Dietary Guidelines

The purpose of this chapter is to help you choose a suitable diet for balance, harmony, and health in your life, based on Ayurvedic principles. Health-conscious people today are interested in the role good nourishment can play in their healing and in their health.

Many have come to realize that proper food and diet can make a vital contribution to good health, while inappropriate eating is often responsible for poor health, lack of vitality, and susceptibility to disease.

The Ayurvedic tradition offers much insight into what food will suit and balance each individual, how to prepare and cook this food properly, how to avoid food combinations that will create toxins in the body, and what eating habits to cultivate—and which to avoid —in order to receive the most nourishment from what you eat. All these topics, except specific guidelines on how to prepare and cook the food, will be discussed in this chapter.

Food Guidelines for the Constitutional Types

What you eat should be suited to your individual constitution. Ideally, in deciding what to eat, you would know your constitution and understand its relationship to the qualities of various kinds of food, including whether each food would be helpful or aggravating to your unique doshic balance. You would have to take into account the taste of the food (we will discuss that issue later in this chapter), and whether its qualities are heavy or light, oily or dry, liquid or solid. You would also have to know whether the food is cooling or heating (virya), and its postdigestive effect (vipaka).

If you are interested, you can go more deeply into Ayurvedic theory in order to fully comprehend these factors. Otherwise, the following charts take these factors into consideration in recommending what foods to eat or avoid.

The charts categorize foods according to their suitability for each doshic type. Here are a few points to remember:

- Foods marked "no" tend to aggravate that particular dosha, while foods marked "yes" pacify or balance that dosha. In planning your diet, choose foods that create balance, and avoid those that might provoke your predominant doshas or the dosha that is currently aggravated or increased.

- The recommendations are not meant to be absolute, but are guidelines. If a food is on your "no" list, that means you should avoid it most of the time, and if you eat it, eat a modest amount or do something to modify its effects. Apples, for example, are quite vataprovoking if eaten raw. But if you cook them and eat them warm, with a little ghee and warming spices such as cardamom or cinnamon, they are fine for vata individuals in modest amounts.

- Keep the seasons in mind. Summer, for example, is pitta season, and it is not good—especially for people with a predominantly pitta constitution—to eat too many hot, spicy foods, or pitta dosha will become aggravated. Similarly, during autumn, when the air is dry and cool and more vata is present in the atmosphere, everyone—but especially individuals with a vata constitution—should avoid dry fruit, salads, cold foods, and other vata-provoking items. In winter and early spring, the heavy, cold, moist season of kapha, one should make an extra effort to avoid cold food and drinks, ice cream, cheese, yogurt, elons, and other kapha-increasing foods.

- For individuals with a dual constitution (two doshas approximately equal), a little extra care is needed, but you can figure it out. For example, a vata-pitta individual needs to avoid vata-increasing foods in the fall and winter (but without increasing pitta too much) and minimize pitta-provoking foods in the summer (but without aggravating vata).

Stated in positive terms, favor vata-balancing foods in the fall, pitta-pacifying foods in the summer. Here are some general dietary guidelines for balancing the doshas:

Vata

50 percent whole grains—whole-grain cooked cereals, some breads and crackers

20 percent protein—eggs, high-quality dairy products, poultry, fish, seafood, beef, tofu, black and red lentils

20–30 percent fresh vegetables—with an optional 10 percent for fresh fruit

Pitta

50 percent whole grains—whole-wheat breads, cereals, cooked grains

20 percent protein—beans (except lentils), tofu, tempeh, cottage cheese, ricotta cheese, raw milk, egg

white, chicken and turkey (white meat only), shrimp, rabbit, venison

20–30 percent vegetables—with an optional 10 percent for fresh fruit

Kapha

30–40 percent whole grains—rye crackers, dry cereals, cooked grains

20 percent protein—chicken, turkey, boiled and poached eggs, small amount of goat's milk, and most beans (including garbanzos, adzukis, pintos, black beans, red lentils, navy and white beans, split peas, and black-eyed peas)

40–50 percent fresh vegetables—with an optional 10 percent for fresh or dried fruit. A daily salad is good.

FOOD GUIDELINES FOR THE BASIC CONSTITUTIONAL TYPES

Note: Guidelines provided in this table are general. Specific adjustments for individual requirements may need to be made, e.g., food allergies, strength of agni, season of the year, and degree of dosha predominance or aggravation. *okay in moderation; **okay rarely.

The Six Tastes

Taste is important and has a direct effect on bodily doshas. According to Ayurveda, each food substance (and also each medicinal herb) has a specific taste. When the tastes are used in the proper amounts, individually and collectively, they bring about balance of our bodily systems.

The taste buds on our tongue are organized in six groups, corresponding to the six tastes recognized by Ayurveda: sweet, sour, salty, bitter, pungent, and astringent. These six basic tastes are derived from the five elements:

Earth + Water = Sweet

Earth + Fire = Sour

Water + Fire = Salty

Fire + Air = Pungent (Spicy)

Air + Space = Bitter

Air + Earth = Astringent

Different groups of taste buds on the tongue perceive taste and send a signal to the brain; from there, messages go out which not only directly influence digestion but also affect the doshas and all the body's cells, tissues, organs, and systems.

SWEET

The sweet taste is present in foods such as rice, sugar, milk, wheat, dates, and maple syrup. The qualities of sweet foods are usually oily, cooling, and heavy. The sweet taste increases the vital essence of life. When used moderately, it is wholesome to the body and promotes growth of all seven dhatus (plasma, blood, muscles, fat, bones, marrow and nerve tissue, and reproductive fluids). Proper use gives strength and longevity. It encourages the senses, improves complexion, and promotes healthy skin, hair, and a good voice. Sweet taste can relieve thirst and burning sensations and can be invigorating. It promotes stability.

Despite all these good qualities, excessive use of the sweet taste can produce many disorders. Sweet foods aggravate kapha and cause colds, cough, congestion, heaviness, loss of appetite, laziness, and obesity. They may also provoke lymphatic congestion, tumors, edema, diabetes, and fibrocystic changes in the breast.

SOUR

The sour taste is found in foods such as citrus fruits, sour cream, yogurt, vinegar, cheese, lemon, green grapes, and fermented food. Sour substances are liquid, light, heating, and oily in nature. When used in moderation, they are refreshing and delicious, stimulate appetite and salivation, improve digestion, energize the body, nourish the heart, and enlighten the mind.

If one uses the sour taste in excess, it can cause excessive thirst, hyperacidity, heartburn, acid indigestion, ulcers, and sensitive teeth. As it has a fermenting action, it may be toxic to the blood and can cause skin conditions such as dermatitis, acne, eczema, boils, and psoriasis. The hot quality may lead to an acid pH in the body and may cause burning in the throat, chest, heart, bladder, and urethra.

SALTY

Sea salt, rock salt, and kelp are examples of the salty taste. Salt is heating, heavy, and oily. Used moderately, it relieves vata and increases pitta and kapha. Due to its water element, it is laxative, and due to its fire element, it lessens spasm and pain of the colon. In moderation it promotes growth and maintains water electrolyte balance. It stimulates salivation, improves the flavor of food, and aids in digestion, absorption, and the elimination of wastes.

Too much salt in the diet may cause aggravation of pitta and kapha. It makes the blood thick and viscous, causes hypertension, and worsens skin conditions. Feeling hot, fainting, skin wrinkling, and baldness may be due to excessive use of the salty taste. Salt may also induce water retention and edema. Patchy hair loss, ulcers, bleeding disorders, skin eruptions, and hyperacidity may all result from overuse of the salty taste.

PUNGENT

The pungent taste is present in various hot peppers (cayenne, chili, black), as well as in onions, radishes, garlic, mustard, and ginger. It is light, drying, and heating in nature. Used in moderation, it improves digestion and absorption and cleans the mouth. It clears the sinuses by stimulating nasal secretions and tearing of the eyes. The pungent taste aids circulation, breaks up clots, helps in the elimination of waste products, and kills germs and parasites. It brings clarity of perception.

On the other hand, overuse of the pungent taste in the daily diet may cause negative reactions. It can kill sperm and ova, causing sexual debility in both sexes. It may induce burning, choking, fainting, and fatigue with feelings of heat and thirst. By aggravating pitta, it can cause diarrhea, heartburn, and nausea. Pungency can also aggravate vata (it is derived from both the fire and air elements), resulting in giddiness, tremors, insomnia, or pain in the leg muscles. Peptic ulcers, asthma, colitis, and skin conditions may result from excessive use.

BITTER

This taste is found in coffee, bitter melon, aloe vera, rhubarb, and the herbs yellow dock, fenugreek, turmeric root, dandelion root, and sandalwood. Bitter is the taste most lacking in the North American diet. It is cool, light, and dry in nature, increases vata, and decreases pitta and kapha. Though bitter is not delicious in itself, it promotes the flavor of other tastes. It is antitoxic and kills germs. It helps to relieve burning sensations, itching, fainting, and obstinate skin disorders. It reduces fever and stimulates firmness of the skin and muscles. In a small dose it can relieve intestinal gas and works as a digestive tonic. It is drying to the system and causes a reduction in fat, bone marrow, urine, and feces.

Overuse of the bitter taste may deplete plasma, blood, muscles, fat, bone marrow, and semen and may result in sexual debility. Extreme dryness and roughness, emaciation, and weariness may be the result of excessive eating of the bitter taste. It may at times induce dizziness and unconsciousness.

ASTRINGENT

The astringent taste is present in unripe bananas, pomegranates, chickpeas, green beans, yellow split peas, okra, alfalfa sprouts, and the herbs goldenseal, turmeric, lotus seed, arjuna, and alum. It is cooling, drying, and heavy in nature and produces a dry, choking sensation in the throat. Taken in moderation, the astringent taste calms pitta and kapha but excites vata. It helps in the healing of ulcers and stops bleeding by promoting clotting.

Excess use may cause dryness in the mouth, difficulty in speech, and constipation, as well as abdominal distention, heart spasms, and stagnation of circulation. It may affect the sex drive and lead to depletion of sperm. It can give rise to emaciation, convulsions, Bell's palsy, stroke paralysis, and other neuromuscular vata disorders.

EFFECTS OF TASTES ON THE DOSHAS

The tastes have the following effects upon the doshas:

VATA. People of vata constitution should avoid bitter, pungent, and astringent substances in excess, because they increase air and have a tendency to cause gas. Foods and herbs containing sweet, sour, and salty tastes are good for individuals of vata constitution.

Herbs and the Six Tastes

The taste of an herb is not incidental but is directly related—indeed, directly responsible—for much of its therapeutic value. That is why Ayurvedic herbs are generally taken in a form that requires tasting them, rather than concealing the taste in a capsule.

There is no problem in taking an herb that has a sweet, pungent, or otherwise tempting taste. But most people, particularly in Western culture, don't like the bitter or astringent tastes, and if they have to take an herb with either of these tastes, they want to put the herb into a capsule and swallow it without tasting it. Since the stomach has no taste buds, when the herb is taken this way, the effects and benefits derived from the taste are lessened, because they are not perceived. When we eat food, we don't lose the effect of the tastes because we have to chew; when we use capsules, we miss the taste of the herb.

One of the reasons the Ayurvedic physician prescribes an herb is to balance whatever taste is lacking in the body. The herb transmits that taste and its effects into rasa dhatu (plasma). Triphala, for example, provides all the tastes except salty, but it tends to yield the predominant taste that is lacking in the body, which for most Westerners is the bitter taste. That's why for many people triphala tastes bitter for some time. Later, after regular use, the bitter taste will have been received into the rasa dhatu, and triphala may taste sour or sweet.

In Ayurvedic medicine, most herbs are classified according to their predominant taste, secondary aftertaste, and "potential" taste. The main taste acts on rasa dhatu, the aftertaste acts on the nervous system, and the third taste has either a heating or a cooling effect.

This explains why it is important to have the effect of taste on the tongue when taking Ayurvedic medications.

PITTA. Pitta individuals should avoid sour, salty, and pungent substances, which aggravate bodily fire. However, sweet, bitter, and astringent tastes are beneficial for pittas.

KAPHA. Kapha individuals should avoid foods containing the sweet, sour, and salty tastes, for they increase bodily water. Better for them are foods with pungent, bitter, and astringent tastes.

Healthy and Unhealthy Eating Habits

How you eat is as important as what you eat. Here are some suggestions for healthy eating, followed by a list of habits to avoid.

EATING HABITS TO CULTIVATE

Choose foods according to your constitution. They will nourish you and not aggravate your doshas.

Choose foods according to the season.

Eat fresh, sattvic food of the best quality you can afford.

Do not eat unless you feel hungry.

Do not drink unless you feel thirsty. If you are hungry and you drink instead of eating,

the liquid will dissolve the digestive enzymes and reduce your gastric fire.

Sit, don't stand, to eat.

When eating, eat. That is, don't read, watch TV, or be distracted by too much

conversation. Focus on the food.

Chew well, at least 32 times per mouthful. This enables the digestive enzymes in the

mouth to do their work properly.

Eat at a moderate speed. Don't gobble your food.

Fill one-third of your stomach with food, one-third with water, and leave one-third

empty.

Don't eat more at a meal than the amount of food you can hold in two cupped hands.

Overeating expands the stomach so that you will feel the need for additional food.

Overeating also creates toxins in the digestive tract.

During meals, don't drink iced drinks or fruit juice, sip a little warm water between

mouthfuls of food.

Honey should never be cooked. If it is cooked, the molecules become like a glue that adheres to mucous membranes and clogs the subtle channels, producing toxins.

UNHEALTHY EATING HABITS

Overeating

Eating too soon after a full meal

Drinking too much water, or no water, during a meal

Drinking very chilled water during a meal, or indeed at any time

Eating when constipated

Eating at the wrong time of day, either too early or too late.

Eating too much heavy food or too little light food

Eating fruit or drinking fruit juice with a meal

Eating without real hunger

Emotional eating

Eating incompatible food combinations

Munching between meals

Incompatible Food Combinations

The shelves of pharmacies and health food stores these days are lined with digestive aids and pills for indigestion and gas. It is likely that most of these gastrointestinal problems begin with poor food combining.

According to Ayurveda, certain food combinations disturb the normal functioning of the gastric fire and upset the balance of the doshas. Combining foods improperly can produce indigestion, fermentation, putrefaction, and gas formation. If such a situation in your stomach and intestines is frequent or prolonged, it can lead to disease. As just one example, eating bananas with milk can diminish agni (gastric fire) and change the intestinal flora, resulting in toxins and causing sinus congestion, cold, cough, allergies, hives, and rash. Such disturbances generate ama, the toxic substance that is the root cause of most ailments.

The following table lists some (but far from all) of the incompatible food combinations worth avoiding. You can alleviate some of the ill effects of these combinations by using spices and herbs in your cooking. A strong digestive fire can be the most powerful means of dealing with these combinations. Chew a bit of fresh ginger (sprinkled with salt and lime juice if you like) before meals to stimulate digestion.

NAME OF FOOD INCOMPATIBLE WITH

- MILK BANANAS

Fish, Melons, Yogurt, Sour Fruits, Kitchari (mung dal and

basmati rice), Bread made with yeast

- YOGURT MILK

Sour fruits, Melons, Hot drinks—including coffee and tea—Fish,

Mango (thus mango lassi is not a good idea), Starches, Cheese,

Banana

- MELONS EVERYTHING, especially:

"Eat them alone or leave

them alone" Grains, Starches, Fried foods, Cheese

- EGGS MILK

Yogurt, Melons, Cheese, Fruits, Potatoes

- STARCHES BANANAS

Eggs, Milk, Dates

- HONEY GHEE in equal proportions (by weight)

(never cook honey) Grains

- CORN Dates, Raisins, Bananas
- LEMONS Yogurt, Milk, Cucumber, Tomato
- NIGHTSHADES (Potato, tomato, eggplant) Yogurt, Milk, Melon, Cucumber

Particularly to be avoided are such concoctions as banana milkshakes and "fruit smoothies" made with milk. Mixed fruit salads are also incompatible. Some blended fruit drinks made with all fruit may be all right, but check this chart first.

Recommendations Regarding Milk and Milk Products

In Ayurveda, milk and dairy products such as ghee and freshly made yogurt are considered highly important to the diet. However, the process of pasteurization, which kills bacteria and other potentially harmful microorganisms, may also destroy the enzymes necessary for proper digestion. If the milk is heated for a fairly long period of time, such as fifteen or twenty minutes, the enzymes will definitely be destroyed, and calcium and other nutrients may not be absorbed.

When milk is heated just until it reaches the boiling point, its enzymes are not destroyed, and it becomes less kaphagenic. So if you can obtain organic, unpasteurized milk from certified dairies and heat it just to the boiling point, that would be best.

Nevertheless, pasteurized milk from the supermarket, and dairy products made from that milk, are still better than no dairy products at all.

Note that for each food in capital letters on the left, the food in capitals on the right is the most incompatible; foods in small letters are less incompatible.

Food and the Three Gunas

The Ayurvedic tradition teaches that food is not only for nutrition, to nourish the body, but also affects the mind and consciousness. As we have a physical constitution (vata–pitta– kapha), we also have a mental constitution characterized by the three gunas: sattva, rajas, and tamas.

According to the Sankhya philosophy of creation, sattva, rajas, and tamas are universal qualities necessary for the creation of the universe. They are equally necessary for maintaining our psychobiological functions.

Because of sattva, we remain conscious and reawaken every morning. Because of rajas, our thoughts, feelings, and emotions move in a creative way. Because of tamas, we become tired, exhausted, and heavy; without tamas there is no sleep. Another way to look at it is that sattva brings clarity, rajas brings perception, and tamas gives solid, concrete experience.

These three qualities are also necessary for the functioning of every cell. Satva is potential energy, rajas is kinetic energy, and tamas is inertia. The potential energy in the cell is awareness; it becomes active due to the kinetic energy of rajas; then the cell becomes inert because of the tamasic quality. Thus these three qualities are absolutely necessary for the psychobiological activities of the human body.

Psychological Constitutions

Indian philosophy classifies human temperaments into three basic types: sattvic, rajasic, and tamasic. These types all differ in psychological and moral disposition, as well as in their reactions to social, cultural, and physical conditions, as is described in the classical texts of Ayurveda.

Sattvic qualities imply essence, reality, consciousness, purity, and clarity of perception. People in whom sattvic qualities predominate are loving, compassionate, religious, and pure-minded, following truth and righteousness. They tend to have good manners and positive behavior, and they do not easily become upset or angry.

Although they work hard mentally, they do not get mental fatigue, so they need only four to five hours of sleep at night. They look fresh, alert, aware, and full of luster and are recognized for their wisdom, happiness, and joy. They are creative, humble, and respectful of their teachers. Worshiping God and humanity, they love all. They care for people, birds, animals, and trees and are respectful of every life and existence.

Rajasic individuals are loving, calm, and patient—so long as their own interests are served! All their activities are self-centered and egotistical. They are kind, friendly, and faithful only to those who are helpful to them.

All movement and activity is due to rajas, which leads to the life of sensual enjoyment, pleasure and pain, effort and restlessness. People in whom rajasic qualities predominate tend to be egoistic, ambitious, aggressive, proud, and competitive and have a tendency to control others. They like power, prestige, and position and are perfectionists. They are hard-working people but may be lacking in proper planning and direction. Emotionally they tend to be angry, jealous, and ambitious and to have few moments of joy. They suffer from a fear of failure, are subject to stress, and are quickly drained of mental energy. They require eight hours of sleep.

Tamas is darkness, inertia, heaviness, and a tendency toward materialism. Individuals dominated by tamas are often less intelligent. They tend toward depression, laziness, and excess sleep, even during the day. A little mental work tires them easily.

They like jobs with less responsibility, and they love to eat, drink, sleep, and have sex.

They tend to be greedy, possessive, attached, irritable, and uncaring toward others.

They are willing to harm others for their own self-interest.

There is a constant interplay of these three gunas in everyone's consciousness, but the relative predominance of either sattva, rajas, or tamas is responsible for an individual's psychological constitution.

In the Ayurvedic literature, food is classified as sattvic, rajasic, or tamasic according to the mental qualities it promotes. In brief, sattvic food is light, healthy food that increases clarity of mind, rajasic food is tempting food that increases activity and agitation, and tamasic food is heavy, dulling food that creates depression and heaviness and leads to many disorders.

Sattvic food is light and easy to digest. It brings clarity of perception, unfolds love and compassion, and promotes the qualities of forgiveness and austerity. Sattvic foods include fruit, steamed vegetables, and fresh vegetable juice. Milk and ghee are sattvic foods that build up ojas and give vitality to prana.

Rajasic foods are hot, spicy, and salty. They are irritants and stimulants, and they are tempting foods (once your hand goes into the bag, you cannot stop eating them), such as salty crackers and potato chips. Rajasic foods also include certain heavily spiced foods, such as hot pickles and chutneys, which stimulate the senses. These foods make the mind more agitated and susceptible to temptation. Gradually, from eating these foods, the mind becomes more rajasic, which means it tends toward anger, hate, and manipulation.

Tamasic food is heavy, dull, and depressing and induces deep sleep. Under that category comes any dark meat, lamb, pork, and beef, as well as thick cheese. Old and stale food is also tamasic.

However, the heavy, dulling effect of tamasic food occurs only when it is eaten in excess.

In moderation, tamasic food is grounding and promotes stability. If, for example, an individual has an excess of the rajasic quality—the mind is hyper and ungrounded and there is insomnia—some tamasic food eaten in moderation will help the person become more grounded and get some sleep.

We can classify food into categories of sattvic, rajasic, or tamasic according to the table on the facing page.

RELATIONSHIP OF THE GUNAS AND THE DOSHAS

Students of Ayurveda frequently ask whether there is a relationship between the three gunas and the three doshas. There is not a direct correspondence, but there is a relationship.

Sattva is present in the doshas in this order:

1. in pitta as knowledge and understanding
2. in vata as clarity and lightness
3. in kapha as forgiveness and love

Tamas is present in the doshas in this order:

1. It is heavy, dull, and sleepy in kapha.
2. In pitta, it expresses as aggressiveness and competitiveness.

3. There is very little of it in vata, but it is represented as confusion.

Rajas, active and hyper, is present in vata and in pitta but is virtually absent from kapha. Vata is approximately 75 percent rajas, 20 percent sattva, and 5 percent tamas. Pitta is 50 percent or more sattva, 45 percent rajas, and up to 5 percent tamas. Kapha is maybe 75 percent tamas and 15 to 20 percent sattva, with very little rajas.

CHAPTER 3

Ayurveda's Staple Food

In Ayurveda, things that we ingest are divided into three categories:

- Poison
- Medicine
- Neutral

Poison is defined as anything that hinders digestion. Medicine is considered anything that we ingest that aids the digestive process. Neutral is anything we ingest that gives support and nourishment without either aiding or hindering the digestive process.

Kitchari is unique because it falls under both the neutral and medicinal categories. It not only provides nourishment for the body, but, due to its spice combination, also benefits digestion. This makes kitchari an ideal food of choice during times of stress on the body, such as during an illness, periods of overwork, or change of seasons. It is also an especially good food to use while on a mono-diet as part of an internal cleansing regime. In order to provide the best quality of energy to your body, kitchari should be made the day that you wish to eat it and served hot.

Simple Ayurvedic Recipe: A recipe for flexible cooking

That's because Ayurveda is more than just a way of cooking -- it is a way of looking at food and life as a whole through the lens of nature's rhythms.

Nature is always changing. If you study what is happening outside your home, you'll notice that not a single day is the same as another. Your body and mind are a reflection of nature, so they are always changing too. In fact, the Sanskrit word for body is sharira, which translates to "that which is always changing."

To become an Ayurvedic cook is to follow nature's lead. That is to say, you should learn to cook with a flexible attitude based on your dosha balance, condition of agni (digestive fire), what's seasonally available and the changes in the environment.

How to cook for the doshas (and agni)

We recommend everyone do weekly meal planning. Outlining the grain, vegetables, and legumes you will eat at each meal in the week puts your mind at ease. However, the purpose of a meal plan is to create a container for your creativity to flow. Rather than rigidly sticking to what you wrote, check your meal plan each night and make adjustments for the next day as needed.

For instance, you may find that one of the vegetables you had planned to cook wasn't available. Perhaps the weather suddenly turned cold and you need more warming spices. Or maybe your agni has weakened and you need a simpler meal to restore the flames.

The chart below offers several modifications you can make to your meals based on your state of balance. However, in order to use the chart, you have to first make a commitment to studying your body and mind. Filling out a daily wellness journal is a great way to begin. Once you understand how cause and effect work in your life, you'll be able to tune in to how you are feeling and what is happening in your environment. Then you can modify your meal plans quite easily.

We've offered many variations in the recipes themselves so you can adjust easily. As you modify these or any other recipes, remember that there is a difference between cravings and what your body actually needs. When dosha is significantly imbalanced, you will often experience cravings for foods that will cause the dosha to continue to increase (e.g., imbalanced pitta will want to add more spices, high vata will crave dry or crunchy foods, excess kapha will only want the sweet taste). But when dosha is just starting to increase, you will find you have more subtle preferences for foods that will bring you back to balance. As you are deciding what to cook each day, be sure you're taking guidance from the right voice.

How to modify your cooking for doshas and agni

To balance vata:

- The best oils are ghee, sunflower or sesame. Use plenty.

- Use warming spices (cinnamon, cumin, fresh ginger, asafoetida).
- Choose heartier grains, such as barley and brown rice, or mix white rice with another grain.
- Avoid cooling foods, such as coconut oil and maple syrup, and drying grains (quinoa, corn, millet). To balance kapha:
- Use less oil overall. Ghee, mustard oil, olive oil and sunflower oil are best.
- Use warming, invigorating spices (cinnamon, black pepper, rosemary).
- Serve lighter and drier grains, such as buckwheat, quinoa or millet.
- Choose more pungent tastes, such as bok choy, broccoli and Brussels sprouts.
- Select lighter augmenting vegetables, such as zucchini, cucumber or carrot.
- Use moderate amounts of salt cooked into food.

- Minimize dairy.

To balance pitta:

- The best oils are ghee, sunflower or coconut oil.
- Focus on neutral or cooling spices (coriander, cardamom, saffron, cilantro, mint).
- Reduce the amounts of pungent, warming spices by 10-50%, depending on your state of imbalance.
- Choose grains that are sweet and moderately heavy (oats, barley, white rice).
- Avoid pungent or warming foods, such as black pepper, moringa, honey or arugula. To balance agni:
- Ghee is best when agni is compromised.
- Use moderate amounts of spices cooked into all dishes. Be sure to include mineral salt and ginger.

- All-in-one dishes, such as kitchadi, restore agni the fastest.
- Choose grains and legumes that are easier to digest, such as white rice and split mung.
- Have moderate sized meals, with not too much or too little of any one thing.
- Include all six tastes in a meal
- Leave out snacking between meals, and avoid tasting when you are preparing food.

Recipe for flexibility: A Hale Pule bowl

Serves 4

Grain (we used white basmati rice)

1 cup grain (ex: white rice, sweet brown rice, millet, barley, etc., or a combination. If you use brown rice, soak for 1-8 hours for better digestibility and faster cooking.)

2 cups water

2 tsp. oil (ex: ghee, sunflower, coconut, olive)

¼ tsp. mineral salt

Here's how:

Rice cooker method: Place all ingredients into a rice cooker. Cover and press start.

Stovetop method: Place all ingredients into a pot and cover with a tight-fitting lid. Bring to a boil, then turn to low to maintain a simmer. Cook for 15 to 40 minutes, depending on the grain.

Alisson Pot

Legume (we used adzukis)

½ cup legumes, soaked overnight (ex: split or whole mung beans, adzukis, black-eyed peas, chickpeas)

1 Tbsp. oil (ex: ghee, sunflower, coconut, olive)

½ tsp. mineral salt

1 ½ tsp. coriander powder

¾ tsp. cumin powder (reduce if pitta is high)

1 tsp. fresh ginger, diced or grated (reduce if pitta is high)

¾ tsp. turmeric (reduce if pitta is high)

2 tsp. chopped kombu (reduce if kapha is high)

¼ tsp. asafoetida (omit if pitta is high)

Here's how:

Warm the oil in a pressure cooker. Add the salt, spices and kombu, cooking until the aroma comes up (1 to

2 minutes). Add the legume and stir to coat. Cover with water by about ⅛ inch. Place the lid on the cooker, turn the heat up and bring to pressure. Turn the heat down to low and cook at pressure for 18 to 25 minutes, depending on the legume you've chosen.

Baked augmenting vegetable (we used sweet potatoes)

5 cups sweet vegetable, chopped into wedges (ex: sweet potatoes, carrots, zucchini, squash)

2 Tbsp. oil (ex: ghee, sunflower, coconut, olive)

¼ tsp. salt

½ Tbsp. cardamom powder

1 Tbsp. fresh herbs, chopped (ex: mint, basil, dill, cilantro, rose petals)

Here's how:

Warm the oil in a small pan. Add the salt and spices and cook until fragrant (1 to 2 minutes). Add the fresh herbs and cook for a minute longer. Place the augmenting vegetable into a baking dish and pour the oil mixture over, stirring to coat well. Add water to cover the bottom of the pan. Bake at 375 F (190 C) for 15 to 30 minutes, depending on the type of vegetable and the size of the pieces.

Sauteed extractive vegetable (we used collard greens)

4 cups greens, chopped into thin strips (ex: kale, collards, beet greens, bok choy, cabbage)

1 ½ Tbsp. oil (ex: ghee, sunflower, coconut, olive)

⅓ tsp. salt

2 tsp. coriander powder

1 tsp. fennel powder

Here's how:

Warm the oil in a large saute pan. Add salt and spices and cook until the aroma comes up. Add the chopped greens and stir to coat in oil and spices. Add water to cover the bottom of the pan to about ¼ the height of the greens. Turn heat to low, cover and cook until the greens are soft (about 5 to 10 minutes, depending on the type of greens).

CHAPTER 4

AYURVEDA RECIPES

We've all heard the saying "you are what you eat." The basis of Ayurvedic nutrition is that we are the result of not only what we eat but when, how and why we eat. Ayurveda is a balanced approach to eating that suggests we eat mindfully, healthfully and with gratitude. Our food should be fresh, digestible, prepared with care and love and satisfying to all our senses. We should eat a variety of foods and spices that are aromatic, visually appealing, and flavorful.

Here's a quick Ayurveda 101 primer: According to Ayurveda, an ancient holistic system, food and herbs are categorized by their qualities, tastes and how they affect our mind-body combinations of Vata, Pitta and Kapha called Doshas. Ayurveda recognizes six tastes and believes we should have all of these tastes in our diets every day. The six tastes are sweet, sour, salty, pungent, bitter and astringent. Each taste has qualities that will either increase or decrease the Doshas. Sweet is heavy, sour is moist, salty is warm, bitter is cold, pungent is hot and astringent is dry. Foods with qualities similar to a Dosha will increase it whereas food with opposite qualities to a Dosha will decrease it and we strive for balance. Ayurveda also prescribes eating these tastes in a particular order, from sweet to astringent (that means eat dessert first!), in order to feel satisfied and digest food properly. Not having all 6 tastes can lead to cravings, weight gain, lack of energy and illness. Got it? Good.

Ayurveda encourages us to eat mindfully, seasonally, organically, and healthfully. The way we eat and relate to food can be extrapolated to other aspects of our life. If our food is filled with life force, or Prana, we will have the health and energy necessary to live our lives to the fullest. For food that nourishes our bodies, minds and souls, try these 10 recipes which follow the principles of Ayurveda.

1. Ayurvedic Falafel

This Ayurvedic Falafel has a twist in that it uses healthy mung beans instead of chickpeas as mung beans help balance all 3 doshas. Seasoned with Ayurvedic spices such as turmeric, coriander and cumin, this dish is cooling for the body in summer.

If you're looking for an Ayurvedic recipe, you will love this dish. I call this Ayurvedic falafel because it uses mung beans instead of regular chickpeas along with Ayurvedic spices. Ayurveda regards mung beans as 'king' of all beans. Mung beans help balance all three doshas in our bodies so it is naturally tridoshic and the best part about these beans is it's easily digested in our bodies in addition to removing toxins along the way. This Ayurvedic recipe has so many advantages, not to mention the AMAZING taste. The added side benefits are huge, this dish is cooling for your body in summer, balances your Vata, Pitta, and Kapha doshas, and includes medicinal spices like turmeric, coriander. and cumin which are so beneficial for our bodies. Make this Ayurvedic recipe to eat well and feel good!

Ayurvedic Falafel [Vegan]

Calories

216

Serves

4-6 falafels

Alisson Pot

Ingredients

- 1 cup of soaked (overnight) Mung Beans
- 1 small onion chopped
- 2-3 cloves of garlic
- 1/2 cup of chopped cilantro and parsley
- 1-2 teaspoons each cumin seeds and coriander seeds
- 1 teaspoon each red pepper flakes and turmeric
- 3-5 teaspoons potato starch (optional)
- Salt to taste

Preparation

1. Some prefer cooking soaked mung beans lightly as they are much easier to digest. The best and fastest way to cook any kind of beans/legumes is in a pressure cooker. You could use a stockpot to cook these beans- just make sure you don't make them mushy.

2. In a food processor, add all the ingredients mentioned above (except potato starch) along with cooked mung beans and grind this into a coarse texture.

3. Mix this coarse mixture with potato starch to form falafel balls.

4. Once you form all the balls keep them in the refrigerator for about 30-40 minutes to set and firm up. It's easier to sauté these balls on a skillet once they are firmed up in the refrigerator and require very little oil to sauté.

5. I like to flatten these balls a little and make them more like a patty, this helps to cook the falafels thoroughly inside out.

6. Take your skillet and place it on a low-medium heat, add two drops of olive oil (or any vegetable oil you prefer) and spread it evenly on the warm skillet. Place the flattened balls and cook them on a low-medium heat. Flip them after couple of minutes to cook on the other side.

2. Ayurvedic Sauerkraut (Homemade Pickled Cucumber)

Unlike Western sauerkraut which uses cabbage, cucumbers are the ingredient of choice in the East. Pickled with spices such as fenugreek, mustard and asafoetida, this Ayurvedic Sauerkraut is healthy and delicious.

Yes, you heard it right – sauerkraut Ayurvedic style! Cabbage has been the popular choice for making sauerkraut for many, many years in the West. In the East it's popularly known as pickles where the food is left to ferment naturally in an acidic medium. Homemade pickled cucumber (you can use any veggie you like) is far better than those at the store. Generally, the store bought options are pasteurized or have added vinegar for preservation. This means they generally don't have the same effective probiotic and enzymatic value that homemade fermented options do. And, most importantly, you get to control the salt and oil in homemade recipes, unlike those at the store that have lots of oil and salt. You know exactly what goes in your pickle recipes and that is priceless!

Ayurvedic Sauerkraut [Raw,Vegan]

Ingredients

- 4 large yellow Indian cucumbers (You could use any veggies you like – carrots, cauliflower, zucchini all go well with this recipe.)
- 4-6 tsp freshly ground mustard powder (you can roast mustard seeds for extra flavor)
- 1-2 tsp fenugreek and asafoetida powder
- 2-3 tsp red chili powder
- 2-3 tsp unrefined sesame oil
- salt to taste

Preparation

1. Wash the cucumbers in water and pat them dry with a kitchen towel. Cut the cucumbers in bite size pieces after removing all the seeds.
2. In a bowl mix all the spices together.
3. In an airtight glass container, incorporate this mixture well into the bite sized cucumbers. Make sure all the slices are coated evenly with this spice mixture. Let it sit on your kitchen counter top for 12 hours.
4. After 12 hours, stir this with a clean, dry spoon. Keep it on the counter top for another 24 – 48 hours. Later transfer this pickle into the refrigerator. The flavors get deeper and more enhanced as the days go by…YUM!!

3. Healing Turmeric Smoothie

Turmeric is an ancient spice that is considered healing and extremely healthy. Start your day with this Healing Turmeric Smoothie that also has Ayurvedic spices ginger and ginseng.

Mmmmm Turmeric smoothie. How dreamy. Turmeric has amazing health benefits. It can help prevent heart disease, Alzheimer's, and cancer. It's also anti-inflammatory! This turmeric smoothie is filling, creamy, and also packed with the good ole' benefits of turmeric.

Healing Turmeric Smoothie [Vegan]

Ingredients

- 1 can coconut milk
- 3-4 frozen bananas
- 2 teaspoons turmeric powder
- 1 teaspoon ginger root powder

- 1 teaspoon ginseng powder
- 1/2 teaspoon vanilla

Preparation

1. Combine everything in a high-speed blender and blender until smooth.
2. Dust with more turmeric.

4. Ayurvedic Oatmeal

Start your day right with this Ayurvedic Oatmeal. Delicious pumpkin and raisins are seasoned with cinnamon, cardamom and turmeric for a healthy and balanced breakfast.

Have some variety in your oatmeal breakfast: go Ayurvedic for a change!

Ayurvedic Oatmeal

Serves

2

Ingredients

- 200 ml water
- 200 g (1 cup) pumpkin flesh, cut in small cubes
- 1-2 tbsp raisins
- 80 g oatmeal flakes
- 300 ml soy or any other vegan milk
- 2 cinnamon sticks
- 1/4 tsp ground cardamon and/or 1/8 tsp ground cloves
- 2 cm of turmeric (curcuma) root, peeled and rasped, or 1/2 tsp ground turmeric
- 1-2 tbsp pumpkin seeds or to taste

Preparation

1. Cover the pumpkin cubes and raisins with water and bring to boil. Cook on low heat for ten minutes.
2. Add soy (or any other vegan) milk and bring to boil again.

3. Add oatmeal flakes, cinnamon sticks, cardamon powder, and turmeric. Cook for another ten minutes.
4. Sprinkle with the pumpkin seeds and serve.

5. Ayurvedic Rose Smoothie

According to Ayurveda, it's not a coincidence rose is associated with love and caring. It balances the sadhaka pitta that governs the emotions of the heart; it's cooling in nature and is balancing for all three doshas. This Rose Smoothie is very simple to make and you'll be surprised the combination of pumpkins seeds mixed with rose brings out a soothing flavor that excites your taste buds!

According to Ayurveda, it's not a coincidence rose is associated with love and caring. It balances the sadhaka pitta that governs the emotions of the heart; it's cooling in nature and is balancing for all three doshas. This smoothie is very simple to make and you'll be surprised the combination of pumpkins seeds mixed with rose brings out a soothing flavor that excites your taste buds! It's definitely a treat to make and share with your loved ones.

Ayurvedic Rose Smoothie [Vegan]

Serves

1

Ingredients

Rose Smoothie:

- 1 cup soaked pumpkin Seeds (you can use any nuts/seeds you like)
- 2-3 tbsp rose jam (recipe below)
- Few strands of saffron
- pinch of cardamom powder
- 1-2 drops vanilla essence (optional)
- Water as needed (to make the smoothie consistency)

Rose Jam:

- 1 cup organic rose petals
- approx 4-6 tbsp date syrup/ Jaggery/Natural Whole Food Sweetener
- Water if using the cooking method

Preparation

Make the Rose Jam:

1. For the raw, more authentic version, you basically add the rose petals and the sweetener in a glass jar and shake it well. Keep it in the sun for about 1-2 weeks stirring daily. This will be nicely sun-cooked and is very rich and robust in flavor.

2. For the cooked version (which is simpler and much faster) you take a stock pot add the rose petals and the sweetener and cook it on a very low flame for about 15-20 mins, adding water as needed, making sure the petals are not getting burned.

For the Smoothie:

1. First blend the pumpkin seeds with some water and later add all the remaining ingredients and blend away to nice smoothie consistency.

6. Chile-Garlic Potatoes and Cauliflower With Turmeric

This dish is filled with healthy spices and flavors. The Potatoes and Cauliflower are cooked with chile, garlic and turmeric as well as cumin and mustard. It's so flavorful and delicious, the fact that it's healthy is just bonus.

This is an adapted Indian recipe. It's delicious alongside some sautéed greens, or with another curry dish, like Masoor Dal.

Chile-Garlic Potatoes and Cauliflower With Turmeric [Vegan]

Alisson Pot

Calories

448

Serves

4

Ingredients

- 10-12 small whole red, or yellow waxy, potatoes
- 1 head of fresh cauliflower
- 2 tablespoons light olive oil
- 1 teaspoon mustard seeds, preferably brown
- 1 teaspoon whole cumin seeds
- 1/2 teaspoon ground turmeric
- 5 large garlic cloves, chopped
- 1 fresh green chili, thinly sliced
- 1/2 cup canned crushed tomatoes
- 1/2 teaspoon salt, to taste
- 3-4 tablespoons chopped cilantro leaves

Preparation

1. Cook the potatoes whole, in the skins, in a pot of boiling water for 20 minutes or until tender. Drain and soak in cold water for 20 minutes, and then halve or quarter (depending on size) to make 1.5-inch chunks. They should be about the same size as the cauliflower florets.

2. While the potatoes are cooking/cooling, cut the cauliflower into 1-inch florets and blanch in a saucepan of boiling salted water for 3 minutes. Take care not to overcook the cauliflower, or it will be mushy and lose its nutrient content. Drain and soak in ice water to prevent further cooking. Drain again.

3. Heat oil in skillet over medium heat. Add cumin seeds and mustard seeds and cook, stirring, for 3 minutes. Remove from heat, add garlic and chiles, and return to medium-low heat. Cook, stirring, until garlic is a light brown.

4. Stir in turmeric and add potatoes, cauliflower, and tomatoes. Add salt, increase heat to medium. Cook, stirring, until vegetables are thoroughly mixed with spices and heated throughout.
5. Add cilantro. Stir, remove from heat, and serve immediately.

7. Ayurvedic Garam Masala

The secret to the popularity of Indian curries lies in the blend of spices called that imparts the unforgettable zing to your taste buds. The word garam means "hot" and masala means "spice blend." Garam Masala is not spicy hot; the heat refers to the Ayurvedic sense of the word, meaning "to heat the body" with the warm spices.

You cannot imagine any Indian cooking without the "quintessential" garam masala! The secret to the popularity of Indian curries lies in the blend of spices that imparts the unforgettable zing to your taste buds. Today, I want to share with you a very simple garam masala recipe that includes only five spices and you can make this in less than 10 mins using either of the two methods I provide. The first method is the easier way which uses pre-made spice powders. The second method is the traditional way that involves dry roasting the seeds and then making it into a powder form to form the garam masala spice mix.

Ayurvedic Garam Masala [Vegan]

Serves

1-2

Ingredients

- 1 tbsp cumin powder
- 1/2 tbsp coriander powder
- 1/2 tbsp fennel powder
- 1/4 tbsp black pepper powder

- 1-2 bay leaves (crushed to a fine powder)

Preparation

The Easy Way:

1. Mix all the powders and store it in an airtight glass container. This lasts for upto 6-8 weeks.

The Traditional Way:

1. Dry roast all of the ingredients in a skillet on a medium to low flame for about five minutes. Grind in a blender or coffee grinder to a fine powder. Now they're ready to use!

Notes

The quality of spices is crucial for making a good garam masala. Most of the spices today are sadly treated with chemicals and unwanted additives and colors to retain their shelf life. Buy 100 percent natural and organic spice powders for best results.

8. Ginger Elixir (An Ayurvedic Digestive Drink)

This Ginger Elixir is an easy to make Ayurvedic Digestive Drink, best to have during fall and winter season. Ginger acts wonders to fire up our digestive system which according to Ayurveda is the cornerstone of good health.

This is an easy to make Ayurvedic Digestive Drink, best to have during fall and winter season. Ginger acts wonders to fire up our digestive system. Good digestion is the cornerstone of health and well-being according to Ayurveda. When our digestive system is working well, we absorb all the necessary nutrients from the food we eat, enjoy healthy circulation and have a good robust immunity to diseases.

Ginger Elixir: An Ayurvedic Digestive Drink [Vegan]

Ingredients

- 1 cup water
- 1-2 inch grated fresh ginger
- 1/2 lime/lemon juice
- 1 teaspoon pure maple syrup
- 1/4 teaspoon crushed black pepper
- A pinch of Himalayan salt

Preparation

1. Blend all ingredients in a blender until smooth.

Notes

For the sweetener, you could even use turbinado sugar or honey (if not a strict vegan). The key is to not to make this drink too sweet, you need to taste the pungency of ginger and heat of the black pepper when you drink this. This is what aids in better digestion.

9. Ayurvedic Spinach-Mung Detox Soup

We all know how stress can take the life out of us! When we start feeling out of control, start skipping meals, have our mind starting to race, have difficulty getting sleep – our bodies are giving us early symptoms of vata imbalance. This is the time to slow down, take time to rest, enjoy nature, and savor warm soothing soups!

We all know how stress can take the life out of us! This is the time to slow down, take time to rest, enjoy nature, and savor warm, soothing soups! The combination of mung beans and spinach in this detox soup recipe makes it a protein-rich, nutritiously dense, and balanced meal. When we eat according to our body constitution and in tune with the changing seasons, the natural outcome is detoxification and feeling healthier. So make this detox soup recipe! Your body will thank you.

Ayurvedic Spinach-Mung Detox Soup [Vegan]

Calories

285

Serves

2-3

Ingredients

- 1-2 teaspoon unrefined sesame oil or olive oil
- 1 tablespoon date paste
- 1 teaspoon fresh minced ginger
- 2 garlic cloves, minced
- 1/2-1 teaspoon crushed black pepper
- A pinch of red chili flakes (optional)
- 2 teaspoons cumin powder
- 1/4 teaspoon cardamom powder
- 1 teaspoon allspice
- 1-2 teaspoons lemon/lime juice

- 2 tablespoons nut paste (pumpkin seeds and walnuts)
- Salt, to taste
- 1 cup chopped leeks or onions
- 1/2 cup chopped celery
- 1 cup cooked yellow split mung beans
- 1/2 cup coarsely chopped spinach
- 1/2 cup diced carrots
- 2-4 cups water or vegetable broth

Preparation

1. Take a stock pot, add the oil and saute the chopped veggies along with all the seasonings except spinach. Sauté for 5-10 minutes. Now, add the spinach and water to the mixture. Sauté for few more minutes. At the end add the mung beans and simmer until everything is well incorporated.

2. Blend to a soup like consistency. When ready to serve, garnish with parsley and tomatoes. Small cubed avocados go well with this soup.

10. Kitchari – The Nutritious Ayurvedic Detox Dish

Kitchari has been Ayurveda's age-old signature detox dish! The word "kitchari" in India means mixture of two or more grains. This dish takes a western twist with protein-rich quinoa in place of white basmati rice, which makes this Kitchari extra-nutritious and flavorful.

When we eat balanced dishes with mindfulness and gratitude, we set up our bodies for optimal health. If you've been thinking about eating the Ayurvedic way, start with these delicious recipes.

Kitchari has been Ayurveda's age-old signature detox dish! The word "kitchari" (pronounced kitch-a-ree) in India means mixture of two or more grains. Easy to make and healthy to eat. Traditional Kitchari is made by mixing white basmati rice and split yellow mung dal. This dish takes a western twist with protein-rich quinoa in place of white basmati rice, which makes this Kitchari extra-nutritious and flavorful.

Kitchari – The Nutritious Ayurvedic Detox Dish [Vegan, Gluten-Free]

Calories

543

Serves

2-3

Ingredients

For the Kitchari:

- 1 cup quinoa (preferably soaked for 3-4 hrs)
- 1 cup split mung beans (preferably soaked for 2-3 hrs)
- 1 teaspoon olive oil or coconut oil
- 1 teaspoon cumin and mustard seeds
- 1 teaspoon fennel powder

- 1 1/2 teaspoons coriander powder
- 1/2 teaspoon turmeric powder
- 1/2 teaspoon asafoetida powder
- 1-2 teaspoons red chili powder (optional)
- 2-3 tablespoons chopped cilantro
- 1 teaspoon freshly squeezed lime/lemon Juice
- Salt, to taste
- Approximately 2-4 cups of water

For the Raw Topping Sauce:

- 1 cup of assorted veggies (colorful peppers, zucchini, onion, avocado, cucumber, cherry tomatoes)
- 1-2 teaspoons curry powder
- 1 -2 teaspoons coconut oil
- 1-2 teaspoons pure maple syrup
- Salt to taste
- 1 teaspoon lime/lemon juice
- Water as needed to make the sauce

Preparation

For the Kitchari:

1. If you are using a pressure cooker you can cook the grains and make the kitchari all in one pot! First add the oil in the cooker pan and sauté the mustard and cumin seeds. Later on add the quinoa and beans mixing it slowly with the above mentioned spice powders. Sauté this for a minute until you smell the amazing aroma. Add water to cover the pot and pressure cook for 4-5 whistles. The consistency should be thick and mushy.

2. This can be easily done in a stockpot; the only difference is you need to cook the quinoa and mung beans separately following the packet directions. Later on, you can follow the same procedure for adding spices as given above.

For the sauce:

Alisson Pot

1. Mix all these ingredients in a bowl with the assorted veggies. For the best flavors to come out, keep these veggies marinated for about 30 mins.

Directions:

Wash rice and mung dal and soak overnight. Drain soak water.

In a medium saucepan warm the ghee. Add the Kitchari Spice Mix and sauté for one to two minutes. Add rice and mung dal and sauté for another couple of minutes. Then add 6 cups of water and bring to a boil.

Once the kitchari has come to a boil reduce the heat to medium-low. Cover and cook until it is tender (approx. 30–45 minutes).

If you are adding vegetables to your kitchari, add the longer cooking vegetables, such as carrots and beets, halfway through the cooking. Add the vegetables that cook faster, such as leafy greens, near the end.

Add more water if needed. Typically, kitchari is the consistency of a vegetable stew as opposed to a broth. A thinner consistency is preferable if your digestion is weak. You will notice that kitchari will thicken when it cools and you may need more water than you originally thought.

Garnish with fresh cilantro and add salt to taste (optional).

Makes 4 servings

*Note: The following spices may be used in place of Kitchari Spice Mix

- 1 teaspoon black mustard seeds
- 1 teaspoon cumin seed
- 1 small pinch of asafoetida (hing) powder
- 1 teaspoon turmeric powder
- 1 teaspoon coriander powder

- 4 thin slices of fresh ginger root

Garnish

- Fresh cilantro (great for pitta—ok for vata and kapha)
- Coconut (great for pitta, good for vata, but not so good for kapha)
- Lime (ok for everybody)

Recipe Variations

Although kitchari is traditionally made with basmati rice and mung dal, even these ingredients can vary. Kitchari can be nourishing or cleansing, warming or cooling, soupy or solid, all depending on the ingredients used and the method of preparation.

CHAPTER 5

Ayurvedic Food Combining

For many, the concept of food combining—the idea that some foods digest well together while others do not—is entirely new, and somewhat foreign. But according to Ayurveda, it is an essential part of understanding how to eat properly, just as discovering one's constitution and state of imbalance is important for one's Ayurvedic self-discovery. Careful food combining can dramatically improve the quality of digestion, support the body in receiving a deeper level of nourishment, and positively impact our overall health.

However, most people in the modern world are accustomed to eating a number of foods that do not usually digest well together (like fruit with nuts, or beans with cheese). So why does it matter? The Ayurvedic perspective is that each food has a distinct combination of tastes and energies—and a corresponding effect on both the digestive system and on the body as a whole. Combining foods with radically different energetics can overwhelm the digestive fire (agni) and can cause indigestion, fermentation, gas, bloating, and the creation of toxins.1 This is why proper food combining is so important. Of course, certain combinations disturb the digestive tract more than others—an important consideration if this practice is entirely new to you. Regardless of your particular habits or symptoms, paying attention to how you combine foods can provide a valuable opportunity for insight, healing, and improved health. Remember, food combining is not about imposing black and white rules. It is one among many powerful Ayurvedic tools for improving digestive health and overall wellness.

A Balanced Approach to Food Combining

It is usually best to embrace the idea of food combining slowly and gently, allowing plenty of time to make the necessary adaptations. Some of the recommended adjustments are relatively simple; others can require a major recalibration in our habits, or be met with resistance. Often, simply developing an awareness of the improper food combinations that you eat somewhat regularly is a great place to start. Notice which foods you combine that may be difficult to digest together, and how often you indulge in them. Become aware of how you feel afterward. Do these choices affect your energy level, your digestion, your elimination, the coating on your tongue? Are particular combinations more noticeably influential than others? These are all important pieces of information. They can confirm the importance of proper food combining and can help each of us to identify the food combinations that are the most disruptive to our systems.

When you are feeling motivated and decide that you are ready to start adapting your diet to accommodate more supportive food combinations, consider tackling just one change at a time. Perhaps you'll start by eating fruits alone, rather than in combination with other foods. Over time, you can gradually progress toward the ideal. While it would certainly be nice to avoid improper food combinations altogether, reducing their frequency can also be incredibly beneficial. If you do find that some specific food combinations are more problematic for you or your loved ones than others, focus your efforts on changing just those in the beginning. The most important first step is to become aware of your needs and your habits; from there, you can evolve an approach to food combining that works for you.

Combinations to Reduce or Avoid

The following list highlights incompatible foods and offers suggestions for more appropriate combinations. It is meant to be a helpful guide, not an exhaustive list. In fact, you may be aware of other combinations that do not work for your body. Honor those instincts. Because this resource is meant to help you determine optimal combinations at a glance, there is some repetition. Combinations listed in all caps are particularly challenging.

Yes, some of these are staple combinations in many households. Pizza and a number of other beloved Italian dishes combine nightshades with cheese. And who among us hasn't enjoyed beans with cheese at some time or another? Then there's the fruit and yogurt taboo... So much for about 80% of all available store-bought varieties of yogurt; next time you indulge in a fruit-flavored yogurt, pay attention to how your digestion feels afterwards.

In addition, there are some specific preparations that are challenging when combined with particular foods.

All of these rules can feel overwhelming, even irritatingly complicated. But, the rationale behind proper food combining really does make sense. Ultimately, combining mismatched foods generates ama , a toxic substance that is often at the root of imbalance and disease.2 But, for those of you who would like to understand a little more about HOW and WHY these food combinations tax our bodies, here are a few specific examples:

Bananas and Milk

Though commonly eaten together, bananas and milk are challenging to digest together because their qualities are so different. Bananas are heating while milk is cooling. That alone is problematic. Further, bananas become sour as they break down. So now our digestive fire has to process a sour substance and milk at the same time. Ever added a squeeze of lemon to milk? Or maybe you've poured a little milk into a tangy, fruity tea… only to watch it curdle instantly? What happens to these mismatched foods in the digestive tract is not much different. When bananas and milk are eaten together, their opposing qualities tend to smother the digestive fire and can disrupt the balance of intestinal flora, which results in the creation of toxins. This combination also frequently causes congestion, colds, coughs, allergies, hives, and rashes.[2] A similar situation arises when we combine any sour fruit with milk.[3]

Eating Fruits Alone

The reason fruits are best enjoyed on their own is that fruit is usually somewhat acidic, fairly simple to digest, and often digests quite quickly. When fruits are eaten with other foods, there is usually a significant discrepancy between the amount of time required to properly digest the fruit versus the more complex food. Inhibited by the more complex food, the fruit tends to move through the digestive tract too slowly and can cause fermentation, gas, and bloating. In addition, the combination typically introduces a number of conflicting qualities into the digestive tract all at once, which has the potential to overwhelm or stifle the digestive fire.

Nightshades and Cheese

This combination is simply too taxing for the digestive fire. A nightshade is a common name for a member of the plant family Solanaceae, which includes potatoes, bell peppers, tomatoes, eggplants, cayenne peppers, paprika, tobacco, henbane, belladonna, datura, and over 2,500 other plants. Nightshades contain alkaloids, primarily as a means of defense against being damaged by insects. The alkaloids can be anywhere from mildly to fatally toxic to humans. As a result, diverse cultures around the world have long held an intriguing relationship with the nightshade family. Some have been used to make poisons, some contain incredibly addictive compounds such as nicotine, some are mind altering, and others create an incredible sensation of heat in the mouth. The bottom line is that nightshades contain a complex array of compounds that, once ingested, lead to a potentially dramatic cascade of chemical reactions in the body. Ayurvedically speaking, all nightshades are believed to be somewhat difficult to digest and to have the capacity to disturb the doshas. When we mix these inherently challenging nightshades with cheese—which is heavy, oily, and also difficult to digest—we can quickly overtax the digestive fire.

Beans and Cheese

Beans and cheese are similar in that they both tend to be heavy and are often difficult to digest. In order to break down properly, they both require a good deal of digestive strength. But, the similarities end there. Beans tend to taste mostly astringent and sweet, can be either heating or cooling (depending on the type of bean), and usually have a pungent post-digestive effect. Cheese, on the other hand, tastes predominantly sour, is almost always heating, and usually has a sour post-digestive effect. The post-digestive effect of different foods occurs once that food has moved into the colon; it affects the urine, feces, sweat and tissues—sometimes even at the cellular level. Two foods with distinct post-digestive effects are typically quite different from one another. This is the case with beans and cheese; when they are eaten together, they tend to overwhelm and confuse the digestive fire. Meanwhile, their combined heaviness makes them even more difficult to process, often resulting in poor digestion and the accumulation of ama.

Ease Into It

Embracing the wisdom of food combining slowly helps us to cultivate a refined awareness around how our dietary choices affect us. This heightened sensitivity can be an invaluable asset, regardless of how quickly we are able to replace improper food combinations with more supportive ones. Be gentle with yourself, progressing at a pace that works for you. You might find it helpful, on occasion, to take a moment to reflect on how your digestion and your overall sense of wellness have changed over time.

Proper food combining tends to awaken the body's innate intelligence, so for most, embracing good food combining habits gets easier with time and practice.

www.ingramcontent.com/pod-product-compliance
Lightning Source LLC
Chambersburg PA
CBHW060831220526
45466CB00003B/1057